NO ONE SHOULD DIE OF RABIES

DR. ASHOK BANGA

notionpress.com

INDIA • SINGAPORE • MALAYSIA

Notion Press

No.8, 3rd Cross Street
CIT Colony, Mylapore
Chennai, Tamil Nadu – 600004

First Published by Notion Press 2021

ISBN 978-1-63873-545-8

Dedicated to the **"Indian Academy of Pediatrics"**,
our mother organization.

Table of Contents

Some Specific Q & As

Plus hundreds of questions you may have in your mind, with my answers on Quora, in each chapter.

- Is rabies infection a death sentence?
- Why is Rabies mortality in India high even when all the means of protection are available?
- Do my family and I need an anti-rabies vaccination as a precaution even when my dog is vaccinated against rabies?
- How can I stay fully protected against rabies at all the times?
- Rabies virus survival outside of a host
- Why do children suffer more from Rabies?
- When so many vaccines are regularly given to children, why not Rabies vaccine too?
- If Pre Exposure vaccination is good, why not give it to all?
- Should all adults be vaccinated against rabies?
- How many doses of Anti-Rabies vaccine can one take during life-time?
- Can rabies be transmitted to humans by consuming milk from infected cow or buffalo?
- Is human to human transmission of Rabies possible?
- Can someone have Rabies without animal bite?

- What is new in Rabies management, an Indian invention that can change the whole scenario?
- Where can Rabies antibody levels be tested?
- How could many countries have more dogs but less rabies?
- Why not Vaccinate Dogs Instead of People?
- Relocating to a different country with a pet
- Oral Rabies Vaccine
- Can India ever be free from Rabies?

सत्यमेव जयते
भारत सरकार
राष्ट्रीय रोग नियंत्रण केन्द्र
(स्वास्थ्य सेवा महानिदेशालय)
स्वास्थ्य एवं परिवार कल्याण मंत्रालय, भारत सरकार
22, शाम नाथ मार्ग, दिल्ली - 110054

Government of India
NATIONAL CENTRE FOR DISEASE CONTROL
[Formally Known as National Institute of Communicable Disease (NICD)]
Directorate General of Health Services
Ministry of Health & Family Welfare, Government of India
22, Sham Nath Marg, Delhi-110054

Dr. Sujeet K Singh
MD,DCH
Director

Direct: 00-91-11-23913148
23922132 Fax: 23922677
Email : dirnicd@nic.in,sujeet647@gmail.com
Website : www.ncdc.gov.in
www.idsp.nic.in

FOREWORD

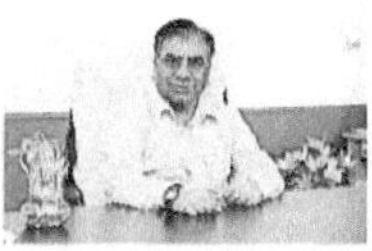

I concur with the theme of the book, "No one should die of Rabies" and reinforce the commitment of Government of India for this purpose. The Government is already working in this direction, as set by WHO, of making the world free of human rabies by 2030.

I know Dr Ashok Banga for many years and his academic acumen. I have read his other books and articles on different topics of public interest.

Our government is also concerned with the loss of more than 20,000 lives every year inspite of having sufficient supply of vaccine and Immunoglobulin and our vast health-care infrastructure. We need to further strengthen the awareness among public and availability of latest information among health-care providers and the commitment for the purpose.

Present book by Dr Banga is an excellent effort in creating awareness as well as making the subject of rabies management simplified and up-to-date for both, the public and the providers. A different way of presentation, the real questions by sufferers and answers by Dr Banga on a famous website, from time to time, make the reading easy and understanding the subject simple.

Hope you enjoy reading this book and learn how can we save lives from Rabies.

22.2.2021.

(DR. SUJEET SINGH)

From the desk of President South-East Asea Pediatric Association (2014) and President of Indian Academy of Pediatrics (2013).

Foreword

It is a matter of great pride for me to write "foreword" for the book of respected Dr Ashok Banga, a most vivid writer on Quora, with 4800 answer-posts, 7.5 million reader views and 12100 followers so far. He is man of utmost sincerity and very vigilant observer – a true gatekeeper of the society.

The tittle of the book – "No one should die of Rabies" itself speaks volumes about his concern about the society. He has so beautifully written and very honestly confessed - why this book?

Reading this book is extremely enjoyable apart from being highly informative and useful. I feel that every person – professional or layman will be benefited from this book. This can be a good companion of every paediatric practitioner and GP and will enable them to answer the queries of their patients in a most scientific way. For dog owners also a separate section is there to enhance their knowledge – I feel every dog owner must read it. Rabies immunization for all and immunization of pets is covered very nicely apart from management and treatment protocols.

We never realise that Rabies kills so many in India – all those die unnecessarily as each and every case of Rabies can be prevented from death. The book very effectively justifies its nomenclature.

Dr Banga has covered every aspect of dreaded Rabies in such a simplified question and answer format that you feel that its written only for you – to satisfy your queries. The questions are very practical and are answered very scientifically with all reasonings and researched evidences.

I have read Dr Banga's first book on paediatric Drug Doses during my PG and since then I have a very high sense of respect and love for him. I wish from the core of my heart that this book really deserves a thunderous success. I wish to thank him for writing this and congratulate him for successfully accomplishing this task and creating this very important book.

Enjoy reading – be inspired (Success story of Goa), play role in combating this dreaded disease and taking a pledge to eliminate Rabies from India.

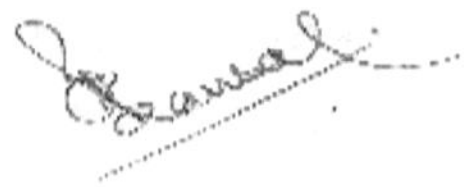

Dr. C.P.Bansal,
MD, FIAP, PGDAP, FICMCH,
President, South Asia Pediatric
Association 2014-16,
Member, National Advisory Board GAVI.
President, Indian Academy of Pediatrics 2013,
cpbansal@gmail.com, cpbansal@hotmail.com
09425111777; 09827063677

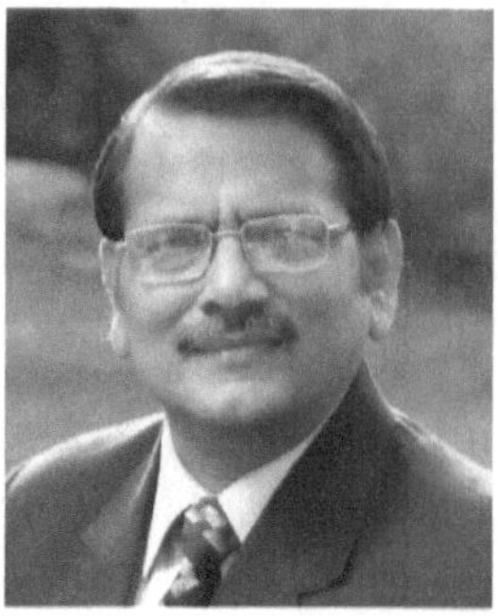

From the desk of Professor of Pediatrics and
President of Indian Academy of Pediatrics, Uttar Pradesh (2010)
Who himself is a renowned author and editor of several medical books.

Foreword

Rabies remains one of the most dreadful conditions. No wonder so, as the fatality rate is 100% in those affected, and there is no cure available.

Yet, the author ventures to say *"No one should die of rabies"*!! Indeed, *no one should*! Only if we have such information and knowledge as has been brought forth in this book.

We have nearly 50 million doses of vaccines available every year against the 6-7 million cases annually. We can afford well to give even pre-exposure vaccine as prophylaxis. Not only vaccines, if we have the knowledge of primary prevention methods, we can prevent deaths due to rabies. This is exactly what this wonderful treatise written so lucidly tries to provide.

Written in a question answer format, it answers nearly all the questions that one comes across on this subject. It is well illustrated with pictures and diagrams. Dr. Ashok Banga needs to be congratulated for this effort.

The book is for all sections – medical teachers, students, paramedics, and the general populace. I am sure it will be an instant hit with the readers.

Dr. Ajay Kalra
Erstwhile Professor Pediatrics
S.N. Medical College, Agra.

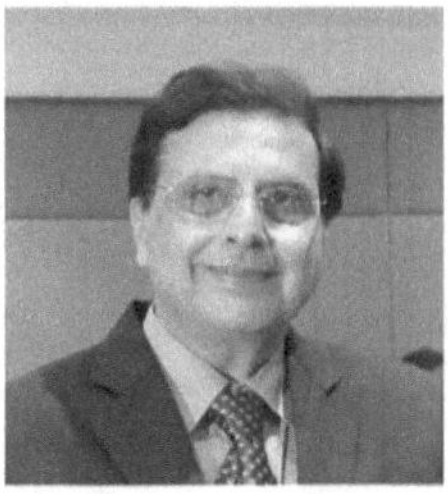

Preface

Why this book?

I had the idea of this book in mind for long but did not find the time. My concern grew more and more for many people losing lives and some unnecessarily going into psychiatric problems for this totally preventable cause. Phone calls from distant places seeking guidance regarding the management of rabies and it's phobia worried me and I was in search of a way to help people in distress. So far, I considered Rabies an illness with straight forward prevention plan but as the collection of questions & answers on Rabies was gradually growing on the Quora platform, it was enough to understand that there is something amiss somewhere.

Although there is lot of literature on Rabies in medical books, there is hardly any for the general public. All the information is not knowledge, all the knowledge is not wisdom and all knowledge & wisdom is of no help if it does not answer someones immediate concern. When people suddenly land in trouble (dog bite or pet animal going rabid), incomplete, misleading or threatening information may lead them to tread the wrong path. Why should otherwise 20,000 people die every year due to rabies in our country despite having almost free vaccination available?

The idea of this book emerged from the following two questions (and my answers) on a famous international knowledge-shairing website **QUORA**, where I used to write on various subjects for the last 4 years or so.

Q.1. Why do people on Quora ask so many questions about rabies and its vaccine?

I am also intrigued with so many questions about Rabies on Quora and why should it be the *top one illness* that has the highest number of questions here. Many are repetitions in different forms but still indicating the need for right information.

Reasons why Rabies attracts so many queries:

1. This is a 100% fatal disease with no cure found so far although this is one of the world's most preventable diseases.
2. There are 6-7 million case with animal bites in one year, 95% of them by dogs. Not a small number.
3. It is common to find stray dogs at all places in our country and in many others and these dogs were never immunized.
4. It is not uncommon to find pets without proper vaccination.
5. Vaccinating cattle against rabies is hardly done.
6. This is not uncommon to find cases even in the USA and many other countries where all pets are compulsorily immunized against rabies but wild animals are the culprits.
7. It is very unfortunate that despite having the most potent vaccine against Rabies, more than 20,000 lives are lost every year in my country. The government provides free anti-rabies vaccine and it is affordable even in the open market (Rs.350 or $ 5 per dose). Because of illiteracy and ignorance people try alternative methods of the treatment for rabies, losing precious time and at times precious life.
8. The problem is of lack of knowledge among the general public and to a large extent among health service providers. Many get confused with changing recommendations and differing advice they receive.

9. Some of the recommedations differ from country to country. Some follow all the recommendations of WHO but not all. Schedule recommended by National Rabies Control Program of India differs from WHO.

10. Sufferers are often ill-informed about who is the specialist of this disease, where to seek help and whom to consult? **No one does in fact**. Doctors at Preventive & Social Medicine really know more of theory but have no much experience of managing patients. Clinicians and GPs manage but they may have little idea of newer concepts and latest recommendations as they see a very small number of such cases in their careers.

11. Poor people in villages and their children suffer more. Their voice is not heard and their anxiety not resolved.

12. This is not a notifiable disease in India and therefore the exact number of cases is not known even to the Government.

The world over, death figure goes above 55,000 each year, India accounts for nearly 1/3rd of total cases.

Stressed out and confused people, therefore, seek information from all possible sources including Quora, that being one of the trustworthy sources.

After reading and writing extensively on this subject, I firmly believe that, when we have easily available, 100% effective vaccine and immunoglobulin, NO ONE SHOULD DIE OF RABIES.

Q2. Many of your answers (disproportionately) are related to rabies or its vaccination. Why?

I am a Pediatrician and Pediatrics is the medical specialty that deals with vaccines most.

I got more interested in vaccinology (before joining Quora) when I got the chance to proof-read a prestigious book on Immunizations, that was published at Gwalior by the Indian Academy of Pediatrics. Here is that book:

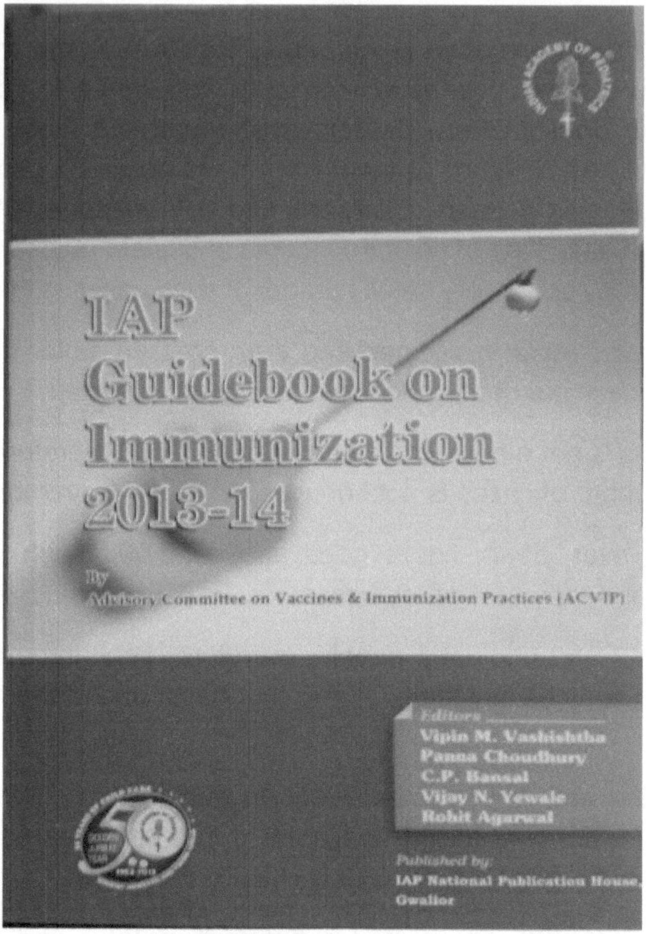

Interest makes one delve deeper.

This also answers 'why me?'

On Quora, initially I answered random questions on vaccinations. It brought more queries and in turn more answers. Somehow questions on Rabies were more and therefore more of my answers. The probable reason is that Rabies vaccination is not done in routine to everyone and every doctor does not do it. Therefore many doctors do not have enough latest information to satisfy the patients' queries, which makes people turn to social media to seek answers.

I have already authored a few chapters on Immunization in Pediatric books and delivered talks.

So far I have answered more than 1365 questions on Quora on this one subject only. There are other authors too, discussing the subject and enriching the knowledge.

With having a collection of so many question that people have in mind and their answers, I thought of compiling all and presenting in a way that a common man anywhere in the world can understand. The present lockdown (for Corona pandemic) gave me this opportunity to complete the task.

In every chapter, I am quoting questions which were asked by the lay public along with my answers. I could get the real feel of people, what they think when they land in such a situation. Additional information has been added from literature to fill up the information gap. The Q & A format will explain almost everything.

I have tried providing all information in simple language. Academic details are purposely omitted as this is not a textbook, not even close because it has none of the formalisms of a textbook. Instead, the book is a bit like a chat with my readers. Its a learning book, aimed at people outside the classroom.

I hope this format interests you and quenches your thirst for information.

I also hope that this book will be useful for those seeking treatment and also those offering it.

Acknowledgement

Time to fulfill any wish is probably pre-determined.

Biggest hurdle in doing something big is our inertia. Once we begin with a clear aim and determination, all the forces come to help.

I had the idea of this book in mind for a long but did not find time and the push. Covid-19 suddenly put a pause on our life and gave us too much free time to complete all pending projects. A message by my friend **Dr. D. K. Bansal** to write a book that I wanted to, became a trigger and the process begun. I am grateful for this gentle push.

Knowledge of any subject is like an ocean that was created over centuries, we have to search for what we need. Quora has been my depository of information, processes, thoughts, and discussions about rabies. I move back to that depository to pick up the pearls of wisdom from various contributors.

First of all, therefore, I acknowledge the persons who devoted their precious time in helping and guiding readers regarding Rabies on Quora. I might echo their thoughts at places. They are:

Patrick Edwin Moran Ph.D. Univ. Penn. & a university professor, USA

Nandita Subbarao writes a blog on street dogs in Bangalore 'Puppy Love RMVRWA'

Timothy Sly Epidemiologist, professor, Ryerson University, Toronto

Liang-Hai Sie Retired general internist, former intensive care physician, Lives in The Netherlands

Sumita Sengupta Dasgupta HOD Public Health, Kolkata

My sincere gratitude to **Prof Ajay Kalra**, a renowned academician and a brilliant author, for inspiring, guiding and reviewing my manuscript.

I sincerely acknowledge the contribution of **Mr Jaydeep Shah**, Accountant General, Madhya Pradesh, for contributing to my efforts in writing in various ways.

I am always thankful to **Dr. C. P. Bansal**, President IAP(2013) and President South Asia Pediatric Association for help in all spheres of this work.

Thanks **Dr. Suhas Dhonde** for providing me his photograph with his lovely pet and his friendly advice.

I am thankful to **Dr. V. N. Agarwal** for reading and correcting my draft at various stages.

I acknowledge the **James Gorman** of NewYork Times for his highly informative article of July 22, 2019.

My gratitude to **Mission Rabies** (a part of World Veterinary Services (WVS), a reputed NGO headquartered in the UK) creating success stories of eliminating Rabies in parts of India. I have included their stories here.

The knowledge imparted by **WHO** resources and **Wikipedia** is helpful in many ways and worth mentioning here.

Wagwalking.com and various other websites are doing good work in educating and guiding the public.

Role of life partner in any project is always enormous and becomes even more when she is also a doctor facing similar issues. Thank you **Dr. Usha Banga**.

Role of children, more so when highly educated, is of a critic, counselor, and composer. Thanks, **Shrey, Sunil, Shreshtha, Pratishtha, Helen and Anaya.**

This effort may be considered a tribute to our long-lost pet 'Annie'.

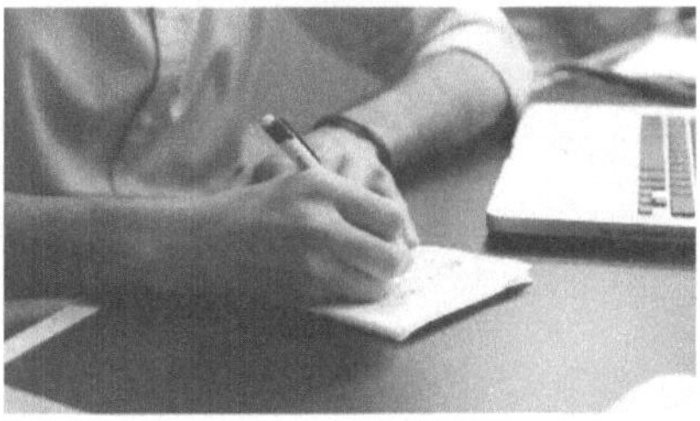

- Ashok Banga

Let us first understand some technical terms that you will frequently encounter:

ARV = Anti Rabies Vaccine

PrEP = Pre Exposure Prophylaxis = Vaccination before animal bite

PEP = Post Exposure Prophylaxis= Vaccination after animal bite

ERIG = Equine Rabies Immuno Globulin

HRIG = Human Rabies Immuno Globulin

M Rab or EQUIRAB = Monoclonal Rabies Antibody

RFFIT Test = Rapid Focus Floresence Inhibition Test

Immunocompromised or immunodeficient = Persons who have lowered immunity due to some disease or are on steroids or anti-cancer drugs

CHAPTER

01

Rabies: Know Something about it

- It is primarily a zoonotic disease (meaning it developed in animals and jumped to humans) of warm blooded animals, more so among carnivorous, such as dogs, cats, jackals, wolves and bats.
- India has 30 million stray dogs which account for more than 95% of human transmissions in areas where they live in close proximity with humans.
- Its causative organism is Lyssavirus type-1.
- Transmitted to man through bite or lick of rabid animal.
- It is the only communicable disease of man that is always fatal.
- Geographic distribution:
    - Some countries have achieved 'rabies free status' by vigorous campaigns of elimination.
    - There are some countries where this has never been introduced.
    - Rabies occurs in more than 150 countries.
- Rabies is potential threat to 3.3 billion people. Estimated death toll is of 55,000 deaths every year worldwide out of which 20,000 occur in India and 24,000 in Africa.
- Although no age is exempt but most common sufferers (about 40%) are children below 15. In India approx 6-7 million animal

bites are reported each year. June, July and August are the peak months.

- Five of Indian vaccine manufacturers make more than 50 million doses of human anti rabies vaccine. This satisfies internal demand and surplus is exported.
- World Health Organization (WHO) wants to eliminate rabies from South-East Asia region by the year 2030 (Rabies Zero by 2030) which is very unlikely. Present corona pandemic has jeopardized all health programs including rabies elimination.
- Meanwhile, the government leaves it to the local city authorities to carry out programmes for vaccinating stray dogs on the street that they are hardly doing. It excludes rural areas, where rabies strikes most.
- Culling dogs is not allowed in India – that is why catching, sterilizing and releasing them back is the only way to curb the disease which is a herculean task.

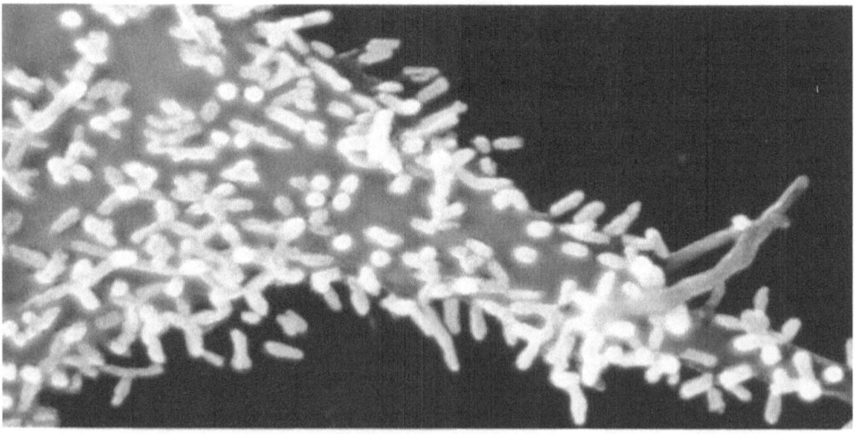

A scanning electron micrograph of rabies virus particles infecting a mammalian cell
(Credit: Science Photo Library)

- Most rabies deaths, even after vaccination, are because of not administering Immunoglobulin. According to WHO, rabies immunoglobulin is undergoing a critical shortage worldwide. It is also prohibitively expensive for many victims in a country where 60% of the population lives on under $2 a day. Only ray of hope is, development of Rabies Monoclonal Antibodies by an Indian company which is safe, effective and economic. One more Indian company has also launched similar product.

- Deeper the wound, more is the danger of virus going into the nerves.
- In rabies, it is better to over-treat than under-treat.
- Experts have shown that annual vaccinations of dogs can eliminate canine rabies, thus stopping almost all human rabies cases. Dog vaccination has eliminated rabies as a major public health problem in numerous countries.

RABIES DOESN'T GIVE LIFE A SECOND CHANCE†

Rabies is a deadly and common threat in much of the world but at the same time Rabies is one

of the world's most preventable diseases.

Theoretically, no human or animal should die from rabies in modern era.

CHAPTER

02

Rabies: Why Should We be Afraid of Rabies?

We must be afraid of Rabies because despite all scientific advancements, means of protection and prevention being available, we are losing more than 20,000 lives every year in our country.

It is happening because:

- Disease once sets in, there is no cure. Death is the only outcome.
- We find unimmunized dogs roaming around the streets everywhere. Children in streets, to and from school are highly vulnerable for dog bites, more so when they have something to eat in hand. They may not report small bite at home and thus may remain unimmunized.

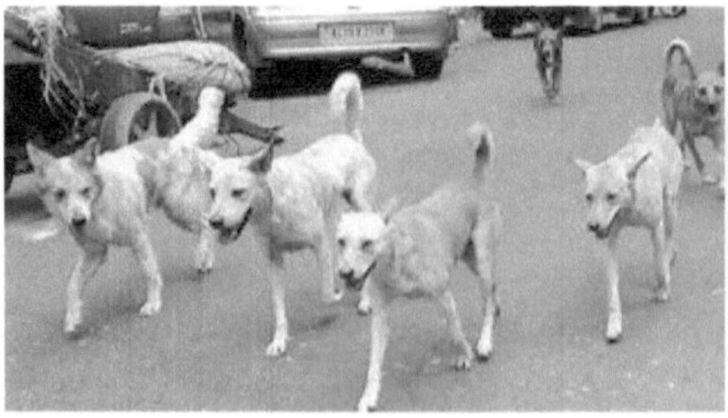

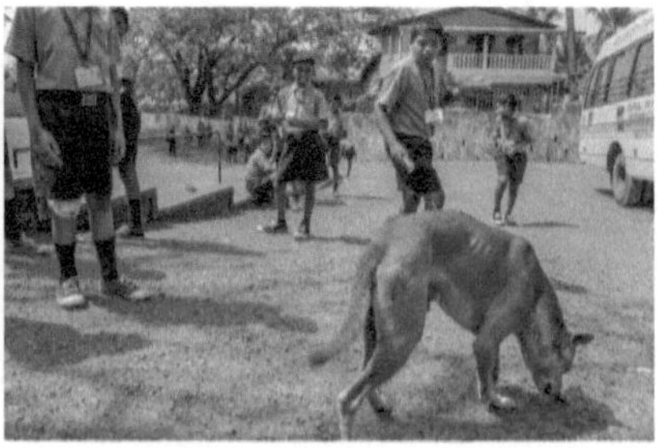

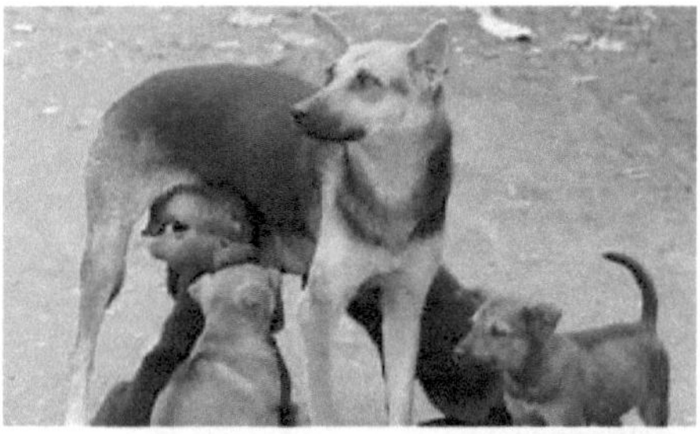

- Many Pet dogs are not immunized properly. Owning pets and not taking PrEP is not uncommon.

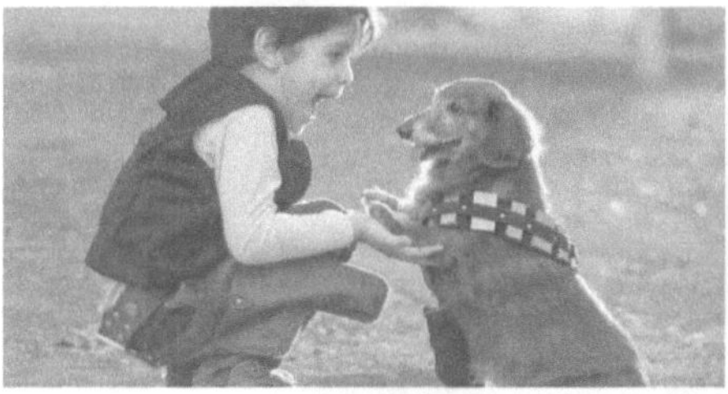

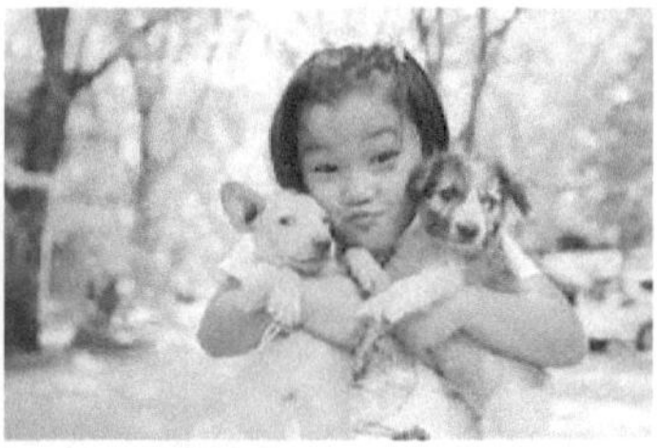

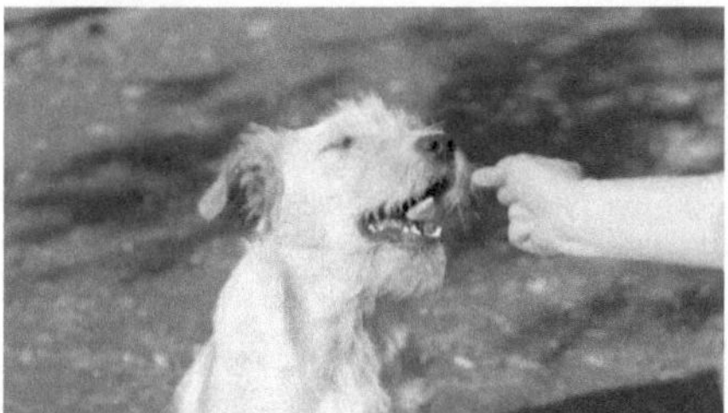

- Monkeys at some religious places and tourist places, snatching food items from onlookers, scratching or even biting at times.

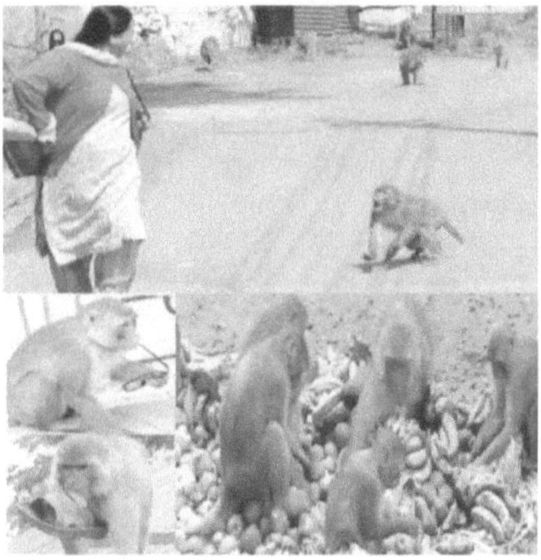

- People working in veterinary hospitals, zoo and in forest without proper preventive vaccination.

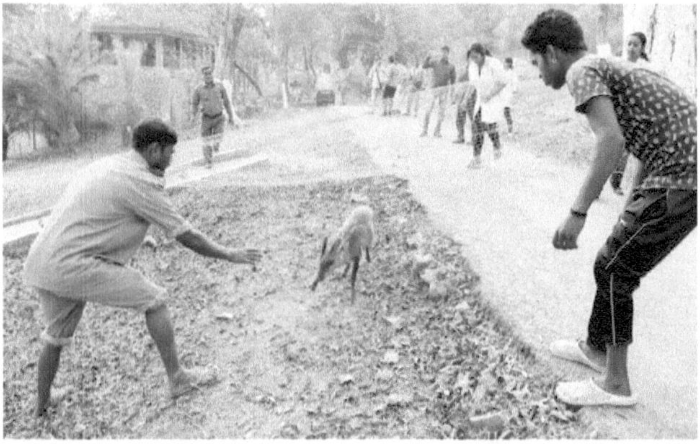

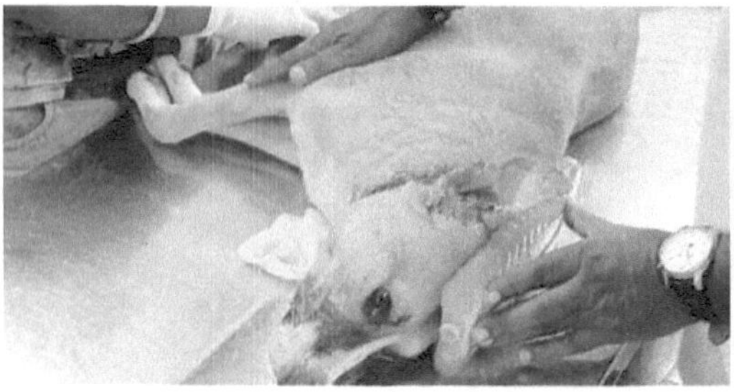

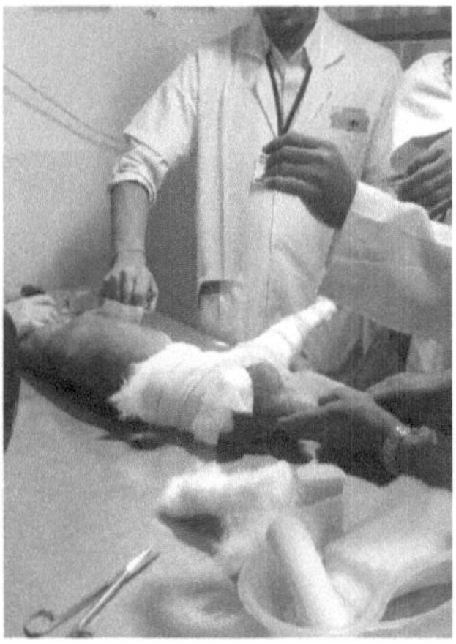

- People owning cattle, not knowing that this menace can affect their flock

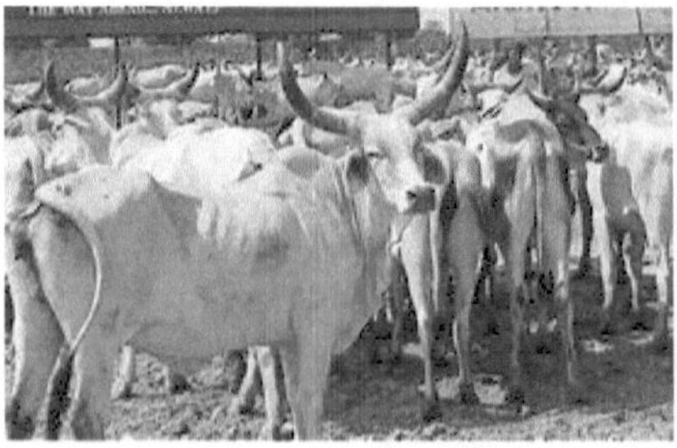

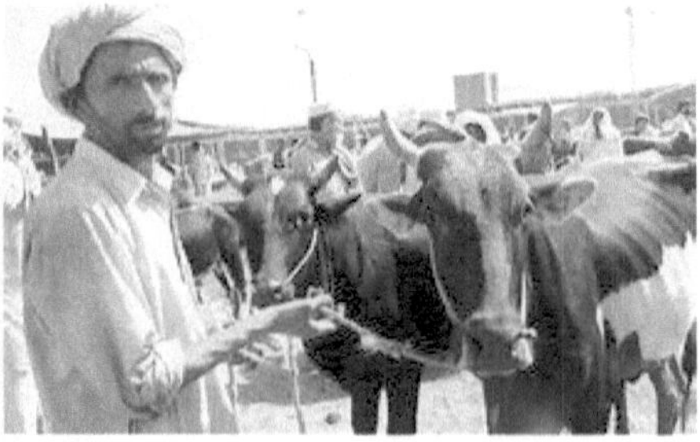

- People and cattle in or near forests are more vulnerable because exposure from rabid wild animals is always a possibility.

- Whatever programs for Rabies control are started are in cities while worst sufferers are people in villages, whether from stray or from wild animals. Lack of knowledge is definitely an issue but more important is non availability of vaccine and immunoglobulin in time.

- Bigger cause of Rabies deaths is that only 2-3% of those who need Immunoglobulin really get it. Cause is not only higher cost and scarcity of Immunoglobulin but ignorance and reluctance of health care providers towards this important life saver. They have to realize it now that cost has come down, sensitivity test is not needed and a better and safer products are freely available.

  Most important should be their commitment towards saving life, when all that is possible.

CHAPTER

03

We Need Not to Fear but We Have to Fight Rabies

Because we have many ways to be saved from Rabies:

1. Soap and water: Yes, this makes the most effective first aid. As early as possible, the bite site should be washed by soap and water thoroughly for 15 minutes. It cleanes and removes most of the virus from the site of bite. Soap can even kill the virus. If you do this simple act, there will be much less virus load that can get inside the body.

2. Vaccine that is almost 100% effective, economical and available easily, makes body learn to produce antibodies that can fight the virus. !00% effective when used in time.

3. Pre exposure vaccination: preparation in advance.

4. Post exposure vaccination: Protection when in danger.

5. Booster doses: to re-strengthen the weak defenses.

6. Protection available on all the fronts.

7. Immunoglobulin and Monoclonal antibodies: Readymade immunity for immediate effect

8. Tests of antibody levels: to guide us about the levels of existing antibodies at a point of time.

9. Ways and means to limit Rabies among stray and wild animals

10. Finally the knowledge of our strength and weaknesses.

What is needed is the application of right information and technology, right in time, for everyone in need.

Several countries have eradicated rabies by practicing above mentioned measures, why can't we?

A combination of all, in time, is the guarantee of 100% safety.

We have not to be afraid but we have to fight rabies.

Because our aim is: in 21st century, no one should die of rabies.

Here are some interesting Q & As that provide information in a way that text-books do not.

How far are we from a cure of rabies after symptoms are detected in humans?

Too far.

In fact, we are nowhere near it.

Any pathy claiming cure is unproven and wasting precious time and money, landing people in danger.

[According to WHO only 15 patients are known to have survived the disease once symptoms have appeared, but all of them except one had at least one dose of vaccine before symptoms appeared. Many of them had permanent neurological damage].

Prevention is what is 100% proven.

Is Rabies Infection a Death Sentence?

No.

Rabies in humans is considered completely preventable if the vaccine is administered after a bite but before symptoms appear. a series of shots after a bite will also stop the virus in its tracks.

The vaccine can be given Pre-exposure too.

When timely vaccination is neglected/ forgotten/ not available and rabies virus reaches up to brain cells, no drug available so far, can save life.

On one side, Rabies is one of the world's most preventable diseases,
but on other side, this is still a
deadly and common threat in much of the world.
This is the example of insufficient human efforts that could have
eliminated
the disease otherwise.

If I get bitten by a rabid dog and don't get inoculated, is it possible I still might not get rabies?

Do you believe in miracles?

Even if yes, how can you be assured that miracle will happen to you?

This is of utmost importance to realize that it is a matter of life and death.

Why should one take chances when life is at stake?

Getting vaccine is such a simple solution, not costly and available almost everywhere.

Do not waste time seeking public opinion; go and save your life.

You are precious for your loved ones.

Do all street dogs have rabies?

No. The one, who develops rabies, has it.

The one, who has it, dies within 10 days (99% of them).

Nature has its own system of elimination of unwanted.

Does rabies vaccine work after bite?

Yes, this is one vaccine that works well after the bite, when offending virus has already entered in the body (but not reached the brain). Such vaccination is called Post Exposure Prophylaxis (PEP).

The vaccine works even better if person is already immunized before bite occurs. That is called Pre-Exposure Prophylaxis (PrEP) and requires less number of doses. Moreover once a person has received PrEP, he or she will not need Rabies immunoglobulin at the time of bite.

If rabies virus is lying inactivated in tissues or muscles for 11 years, how can 5 ARV injections neutralize & kill virus?

Terrorists may be living dormant among public for long time. They are neutralized as and when army arrives.

There was a case where a man developed rabies after 27 years of exposure. Could a vaccine have saved him?

Theoretically yes.

Vaccine given any time before the development of disease provides protection.

This is valid for all vaccines.

How does rabies virus reach brain when dog bites on any part of body?

Rabies virus is neurotropic (attracted and moving toward nerves). Virus initially multiplies at the site of bite, **may be for days**. They travel from the site of wound to the nerves located there, through peripheral nerves to spinal cord and then to brain.

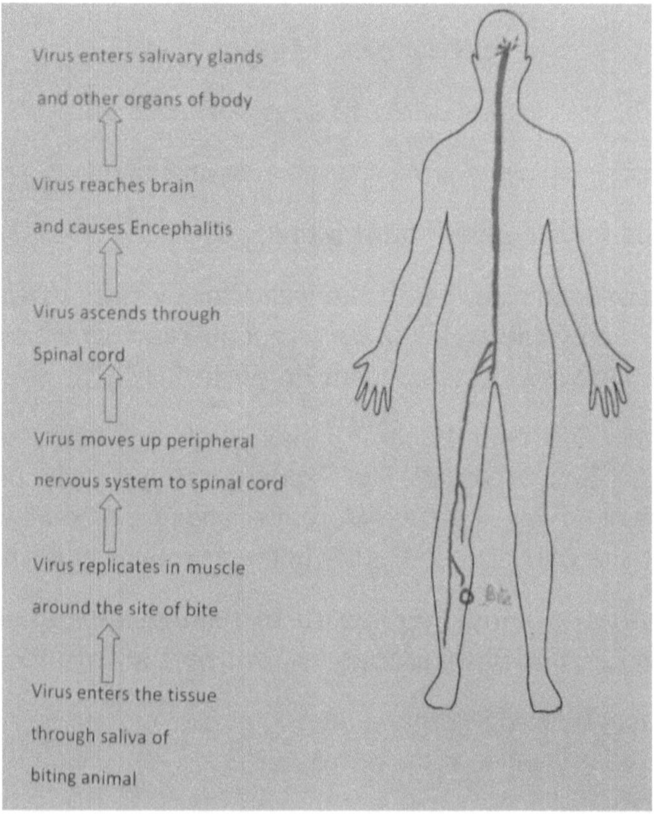

Speed of virus travelling from the site of bite is **3 mm/hour. This slow speed of travel of virus gives a window of time for intervention and that is why post exposure immunization can work successfully in rabies. Remember therefore, that nearer is the site of bite from brain, shorter is the time available.**

Virus multiply in the brain, cause symptoms and travel again via nerve to the salivary glands which are the evolutionary instinct to spread the disease. But unlike rabid dogs which bite, humans do not, so the infection in man is a dead end. Replication of virus in the human brain make patient to behave bizarre where the mere sight or sound of water makes laryngeal muscles go in to spasm making difficult to breath. Hence it is also called hydrophobia (fear of water) disease.

Neurological research has suggested that death from rabies is not a result of structural damage caused by the virus, but rather a result of functional alteration of neurons. The rabies RNA most likely competes with hosts RNA, impairing neural functions. Neurologic damage is exacerbated by the production of certain harmful chemicals (cytokines, and tumor necrosis factor-alpha). In addition, the bodies own immune response to rabies includes the production of nitric oxide, which may act as a toxin to the CNS.

Do vaccines for rabies kill the entire rabies virus that exist in body? I have had 3 risky contacts in a period of 1 month; I just mentioned the last bite to treating doctor and received 4 doses of vaccine. Am I safe from all 3 times exposure?

Yes they kill all existing virus. Your 4 doses taken in the end must have killed all viruses of 3 infection (if at all that was); however, you should not have taken risk in delaying vaccination till 3rd bite.

Why Do Children Suffer More Dog Bites?

Why are children at higher risk for rabies?

Children are most common sufferers of rabies because:

- Dog can easily attack at vulnerable parts like face, head, neck or hands because of their short height

- Distance between these parts and brain is less again because of their shorter height. It shortens incubation period
- Children love to play with pets and even with street dogs and animals also like to play with them
- Children often do not report small bites or scratches to parents
- They often do not know the consequences of animal bite or scratches

Do we need a rabies vaccine for a rabbit bite?

No, not as routine because:

Rabbit in captivity is saved from exposure to rabies.

Rabbit in jungle is mostly killed by the wild animals including dog and rarely survive to suffer rabies.

If suspected, keep the rabbit in isolation, if it dies within few days to weeks if has rabies illness. Then only you need vaccine.

Can squirrel bite cause rabies?

Very unlikely because squirrels are delicate animals and will be killed by rabid animals. Moreovers, squirrels normally do not bite humans.

Still, if squirrel bites and you suspect contact with wild animals, take vaccine for safety.

Is it 100% sure that flies and mosquitoes do not spread rabies?

Yes, the warm blooded mammals can only spread it.

There is a saliva exchange between me and my partner. She was bitten by a dog at that time, is there any possibility that I would be infected with rabies?

Unless she was suffering from rabies at that time, there is zero possibility! By the time rabies virus appears in the saliva, she would be frankly rabid. And if she was indeed suffering from rabies, she would certainly be in no state to kiss you.

Being bitten by a dog does not mean one is rabid. Also, human to human transmission has not been recorded, except in cases of organ transplant. Even frankly rabid patients in hospital settings have not been recorded to directly infect any human.

My friend's wife told me that six months ago a dog which used to live outside their home had licked her wounds on her toes. Dog died recently; exact illness is not known. Shall she take PEP course of anti rabies vaccine?

Yes, I suppose as rabies spreads through saliva and virus entering in body through damaged skin. As both the conditions present here and rabid status of dog suspect, one must not take risk of life. Safer to take vaccine.

My son has already completed PEP (5 ARV course) a month back. He saw a dog near our gate and now he is asking for more ARV doses simply for suspicion and negative thinking. Should I consult a Psychiatrist?

More doses of ARV will not help. Explain him well. If you are not able to convince then go to your physician who will most likely be able to convince him. If he fails to convince then he himself will refer you to psychiatrist.

Sirji, I want your advice and consultancy for my friend from Sri Lanka. Actually his younger brother suffers from dog phobia and in the last one year he has taken 18 rabies vaccinations without being bitten by a dog. Please advice what can be possible harmful effects of taking excessive vaccination and what treatment do you recommend? Waiting for your reply.

Phobias are something which is to be taken seriously, He needs psychiatric help. Vaccine may not harm but is totally unnecessary.

Will a rabies bite look infected?

No. It looks like any other bite.

Can rabies wound be healed?

Rabies infected wound heals as any other wound provided patient is a normal healthy person. Rabies virus does its own work and does not interfere with healing.

Can you get rabies by eating a rabid animal?

Unlikely because

- It is not the flesh but saliva of rabid animal that is dangerous
- Virus will be destroyed by heat while cooking
- Even if you eat raw meat which has saliva also within, the virus will be killed by acid in the stomach.

It can only happen if you are eating it raw, with infected saliva in it and your oral or oesophageal mucosa (lining of your mouth and food pipe) is damaged which is very unlikely.

Animal to animal transmission of rabies may happen this way because they eat it raw and fresh.

Do I need to get vaccinated if I by mistake ate food licked by a street dog? I have bleeding gum problem.

If mucous membrane lining of mouth or throat is damaged due to any reason, it may give entry to rabies virus.

Although rare but possible to get infection this way.

Get vaccine to be 100% safe.

Can you get rabies by simply being near a person who was bitten by a possible rabid animal?

No.

Not even by touching that person.

Is it possible that a dog doesn't die but the person it has bitten dies of rabies?

While I have heard that vaccinated dogs may carry the virus without themselves being rabid (carrier state), I have not come across any reliable research supporting this. Generally an animal can transmit rabies only after it has developed symptoms of rabies. I suspect that the cases which lead to the conclusion that an asymptomatic dog gave someone rabies were simply based on wrong reporting.

Someone could have gotten rabies and reported that he was bitten by a healthy dog without being aware that he got exposed to the virus from some other source (bitten by a bat while sleeping for example).

Second possibility is that dog did not respond to vaccine received.

Third possible reason may be that dog had rabies but no clear symptoms to be diagnosed rabies at the time of bite.

What is the logic behind observing a dog for 10 days after an alleged bite when it is proven by studies that dogs can incubate rabies virus for months?

Is it necessary to take rabies vaccine after 10 days if the dog is alive?

If dog is properly vaccinated and 10 days have passed post bite, you have 99% chances to be safe.

If dog is not vaccinated and 10 days have passed, risk is still there, may be more than 1%, because of variable incubation period in dogs.

And who knows who that 1% is?

Surety of safe survival cannot be 100% if you are not vaccinated because:

1. Rarely incubation period in dog can be longer than 10 days, may be up to 6 months.
2. Dog might have received poor quality vaccine/ in improper doses.
3. Dog could be a non responder.

For fool proof safety, you need to take vaccine.

In any uncertain situation, safer is to start ARV as soon as possible and one can stop after 3doses (10 days of dog bite) if dog appears normal.

Even better is to take 4th dose and complete the course. No ifs, no buts.

What would be the incubation period of rabies if someone is bitten on the palm of the right hand?

Usual incubation period of rabies is 20 days to 60 days but it can be as early as 5 days and as late as 6 years.

Bite on hands or face is to be given prompt care as it takes shorter time for virus to reach brain from these (nearer to brain) sites.

Vaccine takes about 10 days time to induce sufficient immunity, such wounds need rabies immunoglobulin administration for immediate protection. Immunoglobulin is not needed if victim has received ARV in past.

In what volume should a rabies vaccine be given in IM route, 0.5 ml or 1 ml?

This is 0.5ml in some and 1.0 ml in other preparations. As it comes in single dose pack for IM use, you should not get confused with this detail.

Can a 3 month old pet puppy transmit rabies to humans through bite?

Three months old puppy can transmit rabies if infected because vaccination begins after completing 3 months of age.

Is pre-exposure prophylaxis for rabies really safe? What about vaccine induced disseminated encephalomyelitis?

Presently used anti-rabies vaccines in India and almost everywhere in the world, called MTCV (Modern Tissue Culture Vaccines) are all extremely safe. It is so rare to have post vaccine encephalitis that I searched 3 books of Immunization before answering your question and did not find even mention of this side effect.

Vaccine induced disseminated encephalomyelitis was the dreaded side effect of old anti rabies vaccine, known as nerve tissue vaccine, that was given in 14 doses on abdominal skin. This vaccine is nowhere in use in our country. Government of India has already ordered to stop the production and use of this vaccine in Dec 2004.

My friend was bitten by a stray dog and after two days his wound touched a wound on my hands. Should I take anti rabies vaccine?

Most likely NO, because:

1. All stray dogs are not rabid
2. Your friend might have cleaned the wound thoroughly
3. He might have received immunoglobulin
4. He might be on vaccine
5. Your wound might not be raw wound otherwise you would not have touched by that part.
6. You must have cleaned your wound after touch
7. Even if dog was rabid and friend's wound had virus, transmission by mere momentary touch is less likely.

However in case of any doubt, fool proof safe way is to take vaccine. It is not such a big deal.

Do I have rabies? My tiny wound was licked by an unvaccinated stray dog and now it has grown into a big swollen very painful pimple like thing. Also, which doctor should I visit for vaccination for myself, a vet or a human doctor?

Go to a doctor for humans.

Yours is an infected wound that may not be rabies but rabies vaccination is recommended.

Is it true that the rabies virus is dormant in human brain for many years?

No.

Once the virus reaches brain, the downhill course begins and progresses fast till death.

We do not make one odd case an example.

What is the rabies timeline if a rabid dog bites someone?

The incubation period (between the bite and the manifestation of the encephalitis) is from few weeks up to a year, most commonly 3–5 months. It also depends where on the body the person was bitten: the closer to the head, shorter the time taken.

Once virus reaches the brain, the encephalopathy begins and the patient (human or animal) will be dead within a ten day period.

Why can rabies in dogs be cured but not in humans?

Rabies is almost always fatal in all animals as well as human beings. There is no cure available for animals or for humans.

Can rabies virus enter through very small wounds which have developed brownish covers?

Yes, that is possible.

Can a person bitten by a dog take a bath?

In fact he should take bath,

But the site of bite has to be given thorough bath first.

Taking bath is not contraindicated with anti rabies vaccination.

When does a person start sharing his/her rabies infection to others? Does it start from the first day he/she got bitten?

Human to human transmission of rabies is extremely rare. It can happen after organ transplant or after bite by rabid person.

It will definitely not get transmitted by bite from day one. Virus comes in saliva only after the person has developed full symptoms. It can happen while handling a rabies patient, forcefully trying to feed because these patients can not swallow.

Will a person who was bitten by snake get rabies?

In case of snake bite, danger is imminent and that is of snake venom. If snake is venomous, it needs urgent treatment. Forget about everything else and treat this emergency first.

Why do you suspect rabies from snakes? Snake is reptile and does not get infected by this disease. Rabies is the disease of mammals.

Can rabies be avoided by washing with water and soap and applying alcohol if it is just a scratch?

Thorough cleaning of scratched surface is always the first step in the management of animal bite.

It definitely reduces the virus load on the surface and therefore burden on the system to fight disease but there is no way to find out if virus removal is 100%.

After washing, one can apply Povidone Iodine, alcohol, Dettol or Savlon.

If skin is intact, this may be enough. When skin surface is damaged, get the person immunized for 100% safety.

Does rabies spread through sharing a cup of coffee or exchanging cigarettes with someone who was bitten by a rabid dog 12 days ago and did not receive treatment?

Rabies is such a dreaded disease that it attracts such questions about hypothetical scenarios.

Short answer to your query is ‘it is least likely’.

Reasoning:

- A person suffering from rabies will be in such miserable state that no one will dare to share coffee or cigarette with him.
- When he is not that serious, rabies virus might not have reached his brain. In such situation virus is not found in saliva.

- When virus is in saliva and is transferred to other person's mouth, it can infect only if mucus membrane is not intact. Virus reaching stomach is killed by acid.

No such cases of transmission of infection are reported so far.

A dog bit me for just a fraction of second, and I was wearing jeans. I didn't wash the wound (scratchy wound with no piercing of skin or bleeding). I'm taking the anti-rabies vaccine too. Is not washing wound a threat if I take proper dose of ARV?

Washing the wound would have reduced the burden of infection while vaccine taken in time will kill the entire virus that entered in your body.

By taking vaccine, you are safe.

Why does anti-rabies vaccine give dogs and cats a life-long immunity (or three years at least) while a full course of vaccination in humans is only effective for a year? Is it possible that one day anti rabies vaccine will last longer?

As life of dog and cat is not longer, life- long immunity means for about a decade, however no animal vaccine claims immunity for more than 3 years. They do need booster doses.

In humans, lifelong may mean 100 years. Present vaccine is known to provide immunity for about 20 years but it becomes weaker gradually. Boosters help making immunity robust.

A better vaccine in future may provide lifelong immunity to humans too. Scientist are busy searching answers for such problems.

Have there been any cases of rabies infection from virus outside of host animal?

Yes there are but rare.

Rabies virus does not survive out of host for more than few hours (6 hours or so). Hot and dry surface is killer for that and same is with sunlight.

Some of my dog hair came into my food. Should I get a vaccine?

You should get vaccine because you have a dog in your house but not for this reason.

Dog's hair in food are like your hair in food, not good when you look at that and not good when it comes in your mouth although it will not cause rabies.

Could I be sure that the cat is free from rabies if it's still living after three months of scratching me?

You can't be.

Average incubation period of rabies in cat is 2 months. It can be more and even a year.

Better to ensure your safety, although scratch is unlikely to pass on rabies.

If I am HIV positive can I take rabies vaccination during emergency?

Yes you can.

Take a 5 dose course, even 6th dose too.

Immunoglobulin is also indicated if it is bite and not scratch and if your cd count is low.

If a person has stage 1 HIV (window) and he is vaccinated against rabies, what is the maximum effect if Immunoglobulin is not used?

Exact result can be ascertained by antibody testing only.

Can you get rabies from a dead cat?

Yes there is risk in handling the body of cat that died of rabies. Persons handling must have gloves at least.

Same is perceived risk in handling the bodies of stray animals dying on roads.

What should you do if your dog bites you accidentally and you would not have first aid kit?

Best first aid for dog bite is one that does not require any kit.

This is, wash the wound in running water for 15 minutes and clean with soap. Thereafter apply povidone iodine or savlon or dettol if available.

This will remove big load of virus and make onward management more effective.

Should I get the rabies vaccine, given I touched a moist patch of grass that may have been drooled by a rabid animal I wasn't aware of?

To save you from any such hypothetical scenario, it is advised to take pre-exposure prophylaxis against rabies and be tension free for future.

In this situation, only washing hands is enough provided you have intact skin. That will remove dust, dirt and many other contaminants including tetanus organisms.

Why do we need to clean rabies wound with soap for 15 minutes? Does it kill the virus? If it does, what is the mechanism?

Washing clean the wound suspected of having rabies virus serves more than one purpose:

1. Washing removes big load of virus that did not yet enter the tissue. So, earlier the better.
2. Some of the virus may be lysed by soap. Real virus killers are alcohol (70% or more) and Povidone Iodine that may be applied after washing.
3. Washing removes the tetanus bacilli also if entered in the wound through dust and dirt.
4. Cleaning the wound of any contaminants like dust helps early and uneventful healing.

Even if infection reaches inside the body, will be smaller in dose and thus easier for vaccines to work.

Advice cleaning even when person comes late.

My friend's vaccinated dog licked me on my fingers; do I need to get an anti-rabies vaccine?

You just needed thorough washing your fingers provided there is no cut or injury on skin surface.

Why isn't the rabies vaccine given once after the symptoms appear?

Symptoms appear when disease is established and then it is of no help. Vaccine works for prevention and not after the process has completed.

So, vaccine has no use once disease is manifesting.

In fact all the vaccines work before any vaccine preventable disease sets in, human body takes some time to develop antibody against the disease. That is why vaccines of most of widly prevalent diseases are given before any body gets infection of those diseases.

I am sure you are well aware of national immunation program.

Do antibodies against rabies reach the brain, eyes, and muscles after vaccination? Is each and every part of the body protected after vaccination?

After vaccination, within few days, the body defense system start producing antibodies. Amount and duration that it is produced is decided/influenced by body's assessment of the threat. Antibodies thus produced start circulating in blood. Where ever the blood has access, antibodies reach. Hope it answers your query.

Once rabies virus is inside brain cells, where antibodies probably do not reach, it is dreaded because the disease process has started and vaccination does not help now. Hence vaccinate as quickly as possible.

Bitten by an unknown dog at 15 weeks of pregnancy and recovering from a viral illness, will the rabies vaccine and HRIG work effectively?

Remember that giving vaccine and HRIG is **not optional in any situation when life is at stake.**

Even if effect is slightly reduced due to any reason, it will definitely be better than not giving at all.

I request all of you to please refrain from taking advice from random people and from unknown faces on social media. DO NOT WASTE precious time and better be with your doctor who can assess the ground situation.

I read that in Rabies, the onset of symptoms depends upon the distance of bite from the CNS. Why is it so?

This is because rabies develops when virus reaches the brain, travelling from peripheral nerves towards center at a speed of about 3 mm per hour. So more the distance from brain, more time will it take. Bites on face and hands are serious as hands are highly innervated and near to brain.

Does dogs' saliva shed the rabies virus before the dogs show symptoms?

Yes.

Saliva of dog contains rabies virus almost 10 days before you can suspect the dog to be rabid. Rarely this period is much longer.

It means that appearance and behavior of dog can be misleading. Taking precaution is always best option in case of rabies.

Can rabies virus survive on contaminated surfaces under sunlight?

Yes, but for few minutes to few hours, not more than 6, depending on the intensity of light and heat.

Can the rabies virus survive on a bar of soap?

It will be ineffective within minutes because of the alkaline medium and will be lysed soon by the action of soap material.

Can the rabies virus survive in a Pepsi drink and be infectious?

No virus can survive in Pepsi or similar drinks because of their acidic nature (ph 2.5) and high sugars.

How long does the rabies virus live in normal drinking water? What is the viability of rabies virus in water such as tap water?

Rabies virus may survive in water, depending on temperature, from few hours to a day.

If you think of water supply contamination by rabies saliva, you suspect many things.

Since you have asked, let us discuss this hypothetical scenario.

Even if we presume drinking water to be infected with rabid dog's saliva, it will not pose risk to almost anyone because:

1. Dilution reduces virus load.
2. High or very low temperature of water reduces virus count.
3. Virus may be destroyed in water after some time.
4. Chlorination kills virus faster.
5. Even when virus survive in water and reach human body in effective numbers will not cause Rabies if skin is intact.
6. If ingested, acid in stomach will kill all the viruses.

Does chlorine used in water treatment (in the US) deactivate the rabies virus?

Rabies virus is very fragile once out of the saliva or tissue of rabid animals. Chlorine in water fastens its decay.

Is the rabies virus killed in the washing machine?

Detergent in washing machine as well as temperature of water will kill the virus within minutes.

How long can the rabies virus survive on a dog's hair?

Can you get rabies from touching an object a rabid animal might have drooled on?

Does an animal that is infected with rabies have to bite you to transfer the disease or can it be passed through contact with that animal's saliva?

If dry saliva with rabies penetrates my skin through a wound, is there a risk?

There are many more such questions for which following interesting article may provide answers:

Rabies Virus Survival Outside of Host

BY SCOTT WEESE ON JULY 9, 2012 POSTED IN DOGS

I've had a run on questions about survival of rabies virus outside the body. The topic comes up periodically with respect to touching road kill or veterinary clinic personnel working with animals that have been attacked by an unknown animal. The case of three people who developed rabies after taking care of a sheep that had been attacked by a rabid animal, probably through contact with saliva from the rabid animal on the sheep's coat coming into contact with broken skin on their hands, shows the potential risk. An important part of assessing the risk is understanding how long the virus lives outside the body.

Some viruses are very hardy and can live for weeks or even years outside the body. Parvovirus and norovirus are classic examples of this type. Some viruses, like HIV, die very quickly in the environment. Part of this relates to whether they are "enveloped" or "non-enveloped" viruses. Enveloped viruses have a coating that is susceptible to damage from environmental effects, disinfectants and other challenges. Damaging this coating kills the virus. Non-enveloped viruses don't have that susceptible coating and that is in part why they are so much hardier.

Fortunately, rabies is an enveloped virus, and it doesn't like being outside of a mammal's body. **Data on rabies virus survival are pretty limited**, since it's not an easy thing to assess. To look at rabies virus survival, you have to grow the virus, expose it to different environmental conditions, then see if it is still able to infect a mammal or a tissue culture. We can do this easily with bacteria, but growing viruses is more work, especially a dangerous virus such as rabies virus.

I can only find one study that has looked at rabies virus survival (and I can only read the abstract since the rest of the paper is in Czech). The study (*Matouch et al, Vet Med (Praha) 1987*) involved testing of rabies virus from the salivary gland of a naturally infected fox. They exposed the virus to different conditions and used two methods to look at the infectivity of the virus.

- When the virus was spread in a thin layer onto surfaces like glass, metal or leaves, the longest survival was 144 hours at 5 degrees C (that's ~ 41F).
- At 20C (68F), the virus was infective for 24h on glass and leaves and 48h on metal.
- At 30C (86F), the virus didn't last long, being inactivated within 1.5h with exposure to sunlight and 20h without sunlight.

So, rabies virus can survive for a while outside the body. Temperature, humidity, sunlight exposure and surface type all probably play important roles, but in any particular situation you can never make a very accurate prediction of the virus's survival beyond "*it will survive for a while, but not very long*."

From a practical standpoint, it just reinforces some common themes:

- People should avoid contact with dead or injured animals.
- Veterinary personnel or pet owners dealing with a pet that has been attacked by another animal should wear gloves,

wash their hands and take particular care if they have damaged skin.

- People who are at higher than normal risk of being exposed to potentially rabies-contaminated surfaces should be vaccinated against rabies.(Pre exposure prophylaxis)

Is the rabies vaccine dangerous for a person with seizures?

No.

There is no mention of any seizure related side effects of this vaccine in the literature.

Why does my doctor suggest me for TT injection and 5 vaccines of rabies in the case of rat bites?

Domestic rats are not usually carrying rabies but wild rats may.

May be your doctor is trying to be on safer side for you.

Can an asthma patient inhale from a salbutamol inhaler during the course of an anti-rabies vaccine?

Yes. That is not contraindicated.

Do people who contact rabies really bark like a dog?

No. Not at all.

They develop fear of water in final stage of disease. This is called hydrophobia.

Can I exercise 25 hours after my rabies shot?

Yes, you can.

A dog scratched me. It is 3 months old, and had a vaccination just 3 days ago. Do I need to go for an anti-tetanus shot?

Tetanus and rabies are two different entities and either of two can happen separately or together in such circumstances. Be careful for both.

If you have not received tetanus shot in last 10 years, go for it.

Can lack of sleep and anxiety reduce the effectiveness of rabies vaccines?

Probably not but still remember that if anxiety and lack of sleep continues for long time, it may weaken immunity to everything.

Can I get rabies if a person bites me?

In theory yes if the person is infected with rabies virus. In real life, it rarely happens.

For this very reason, taking care of infected person becomes very risky for family members and they are to be shifted to hospital and that too in isolation ward. you can get tetanus after human bite.

In such situation of human bite, the same is the management as for dog bite.

How can I know for sure that the dog that bit me didn't have rabies?

Only sure way is to test the brain tissue of dog for the presence of virus. For this, dog has to be killed.

Another way is to test antibody in dog's blood which takes time.

Third evidence is the proof of vaccination of dog, however not 100% reliable for various reasons discussed elsewhere in this book.

Therefore better is to go for vaccination in any doubtful situation because that only can guarantee you 100% protection.

Will I get rabies if I ate food that was contaminated by a monkey (possibly touched)? I've had the vaccination 2 months ago.

No, you will not because

- You are vaccinated against rabies
- Monkey may not be infected.
- Even if infected, will not transmit by touching the food.

- Even if rabies virus is present in food, will be killed by acid in stomach. Only risk is if infected food comes in contact with damaged mucous lining before reaching stomach.

What should we do when our pet dog bites us when both he and we are vaccinated?

If you are concerned about rabies, you are on safer side.

For that matter, this is the best situation when both are vaccinated.

Only proper wound cleaning and wound care is what you require.

Do not forget the date of last tetanus vaccination. Go for it if you received it 10 years back.

If I got bit by a healthy unvaccinated dog, do I still need to get anti-rabies vaccine?

Healthy does not mean having no rabies virus in the body.

Unvaccinated mean that there is definite risk.

Better go for vaccination to be on safer side.

How deep does a dog bite have to be to get rabies?

Depth is not important. Any injury to skin, even superficial that gets access to virus to reach inside is important. Oozing of blood is not necessary.

Same stands true for Tetanus also.

Do I continue breastfeeding for my baby right after I took a booster vaccine for anti-rabies?

Yes you can.

You should have no doubt in this considering the fact that this vaccine can be given in pregnancy.

What are the chances of getting rabies via sneezing of a puppy which was adopted from shelter, and was sick and then dies?

A human can catch Rabies when saliva of a rabid dog reaches in some depth of skin and then in to blood.

In present scenario, there are many points against spread of rabies this way:

- Puppy must have been taken care in shelter to not have rabies.
- Sneeze may spread nasal secretions and not saliva
- Even if it is saliva of rabid animal, it can't enter skin unless skin is damaged. No bite-no risk of skin damage (unless it was damaged already).
- Once you washed clean the skin, risk is almost over, if at all it was.
- Cause of death should be ascertained by doing post mortem.

If a dog lives 6 months after biting someone, will it have rabies?

99% chances are that such dog does not have rabies.

It is very rare but possible for dog to have rabies that manifests late (long incubation period).

A dog bit me. Which comes first, dog manifesting rabies symptoms or human manifesting rabies symptoms? The dog is still alive and healthy after 4 years. I've been told the dog could possibly just incubating rabies. I only had 3 out of 5 shots.

Interesting and more of a theoretical question.

It does not normally happen or you have unnecessary fear.

Rabid dog dies in 10 days in 99% of the cases. A dog living normally for 4 years with rabies is extremely rare.

A human not exhibiting rabies symptom for 4 years after dog bite is another rarity.

Hope you can understand that having 2 such inter-related rarities at a time is almost impossible.

In simple terms it means that dog was not rabid to begin with and/ or 3 doses of ARV that you took were enough.

Now this is the time to forget that bad day or else take 2 booster doses to assure yourself 100% safety.

If rabies saliva is dry then you pour a 70% solution alcohol on it, will it kill the virus, inactivate it, or will it still be infectious?

On drying of infected saliva rabies virus is killed within 1–4 hours, depending on temperature.

If you pour 70% alcohol over it, virus is killed within few minutes.

Hope you cleaned the scratch properly.

A street dog had accidentally scratched me while I was feeding him. It was a minor one. I had already taken 3 rabies vaccines. The dog is still alive after about 15 days so should I take the last two remaining vaccines or should I stop the vaccines?

You may stop at 3. If you can take 4th dose, it will complete PEP as course is of 4 doses now (as per WHO) and not of 5.

Is there any need to take tetanus after being dog bitten?

Dog bite makes a wound or breach in skin. This can give entry to not only rabies virus present in dog's saliva but to tetanus bacilli that may be present on skin surface. One may be protected from rabies by its vaccine but may die of tetanus if not immunized against tetanus.

If last dose of tetanus vaccine was taken more than 10 years back, it has to be given now.

If a dog scratches me, on that day I scratch my sister before vaccination, can it be possible to transmit rabies virus to her?

No.

Dog scratching you does not mean you develop rabies immediately.

Even when one has rabies, cannot transmit it to others merely by scratching.

I had a dog bite a few months ago. I had a vaccine but skipped the 4th and 5th dose. Is it a serious problem?

Time will answer.

If dog was not rabid, you laugh your way and consider your imperfection as your smartness. You will think that all this science is nonsense and doctors push 5 doses unnecessarily just to make money.

If that dog was rabid and incomplete immunization fails to protect you, you may never be seen on Quora.

Still, there are chances that even 3 doses provide you reasonable immunity to win over rabies.

One must take the recommendations seriously when life is at stake.

Does taking antihistamines (like cetrizine) during the course of anti-rabies vaccine affect the efficacy of the vaccine?

No.

If you are bit by someone else's dog and the owner does not have paperwork for rabies vaccination, should you always get a vaccine in that case?

Yes, that is the safest way.

In some of the countries, where not immunizing pets is illegal, you may verify pet's immunization from vets or from other concerned authorities.

How do you medically treat the survivors of a tiger bite? In addition to normal care, are there any recommendations for anti-rabies?

Yes, anti rabies is recommended for all wild warm blooded animal bites. In fact people living in vicinity of forest, and zookeepers are advised to receive PrEP.

How long does my body continue to produce antibodies for a rabies vaccine?

Throughout life but at different pace.

Antibody production increases on stimulation by booster dose and then gradually come down with time but not to zero.

Does eating meat and eggs have an effect when I am getting a shot of rabies vaccine?

Diet has no specific role in antibody production.

Can I take amitriptyline 10 mg (SSRI anti-depressant medication) while taking an anti-rabies vaccine?

Yes if situation demands.

What happens after an untreated bite from a rabid animal?

One develops Rabies.

Since there is no cure for rabies, you can understand what will happen and it happens fast.

If a dog is not vaccinated, but the dog was also not bitten by any other dog or got scratch by any dog, is it possible for the dog to develop rabies without any physical contact from any dog?

Usual way of transmission of disease is by means of bite or scratch from another rabid dog or animal. Congenital (since birth) rabies is rare and in that case dog will die soon.

While taking a rabies vaccine, is there any problem having sex?

No problem as rabies does not spread through this route.

The person having full blown disease of rabies will not be in mental as well physical state to think of sex.

Moreover most of the people taking vaccine have not essentially acquired rabies infection, it is a probability.

What is the risk of rabies having sex with a person who was bitten by a definitely rabid dog? Should I take vaccine?

Theoratically, there is no risk this way as rabies virus multiplies at the site of bite and travels to brain through nerves and there is no viremia in other body tissues and fluids except probably in terminal stage.

Still, we do not find exact answer to this risk in literature.

In such situation therefore, safer will be to take a course of Post-exposure vaccination.

Should all adults get a rabies vaccine?

It depends on which country you live and what is your profession.

If you live in a country where rabies has been eradicated, no one will receive Pr EP (pre exposure prophylaxis).

Only if some body gets bitten by wild animal, will be given PEP (post exposure prophylaxis).

Ideally in high risk countries, all adults and children should be vaccinated. But the reasons it is mostly given post exposure are:

- Rabies incubation period is mostly longer that gives time to prevent it after exposure
- Risk of rabies is not high at many places
- Preventing contact with animals that can spread rabies is possible to large extent
- Cost of prevention is reasonably high and universal prevention is thus a phenomenal task. Every Government calculates such cost-benefit ratio before adding any vaccine in their national program

However, as middle path, all persons at high risk of exposure are advised to get pre exposure vaccination and rest can take it post exposure whenever needed.

At the same time, if some adult or family thinks of pre exposure vaccination at their own cost, they are welcome to do so.

I have rabies symptoms for 60 days. Is it possible?

Unlikely.

Rabies generally does not give that much time once infected and without vaccination.

What if dog bites me through my clothes and I could change only after reaching home. Should I discard my clothes?

Change the clothes as soon as possible. Wash the affected skin with soap and water thoroughly. Clothes probably saved you to some extent.

Virus is in saliva, if at all present, will not survive for long time on dry surface of clothes, not more than few hours. In sunlight, sterilization is even faster. When washed with soap water, risk is eliminated almost perfectly. Keeping clothes in sunlight or Ironing will make clothes 100% sterilized from rabies virus. No need to discard.

If infected surface comes in touch with broken skin (abrasion or wound), there is risk of rabies virus transmission. On intact skin it does no harm.

A dog bit me for just a fraction of second and I wore jeans. I could not wash the wound. Is not washing the wound a threat if I take proper dose of ARV?

Washing the wound would have reduced the number of virus while vaccine taken in time will kill the entire virus that entered in your body. So, no threat.

A dog bit me 15 yrs ago, and then I got vaccinated within time. Then I got bitten again by another dog 12 years ago, this time no injection. I'm healthy now, but have anxiety due to fear of rabies. Should I be worried about rabies now?

Most likely you are safe as 12 years have passed.

You did not take vaccine 2nd time because there must have been points in favor of your decision.

If you still have fear of rabies, remedy is not difficult. Take two booster doses of vaccine even now and get rid of this anxiety.

Can Indian bats carry rabies? As I received a drop of water like something on my face from a tree, so could it be bat saliva? Two ARV boosters were taken 5 days back, so should I take vaccines again?

You do not need vaccination again because:

1. Bats in India are not found infected
2. Liquid that fell on your face may not be saliva of bat
3. Even if it was saliva, once your skin is intact, there is no risk. Cleaning further reduces the risk.
4. You are already vaccinated.

You are safe.

Previously, immunity for rabies vaccine used to be at least for 1 year but now it has been reduced to only 3 months by the WHO. Why? Is the present vaccine compared to previously used vaccines less effective?

Immunity by present vaccines is for 10–20 years.

Booster is recommended **as a safeguard** for the possibility of **probable decline** in immune levels in 3 months.

Can a person be cured by rabies vaccination after 10 days?

Cured of what?

No, it does not cure rabies; nothing else does.

Vaccine prevents the development of disease once the person is infected, provided it is given in time.

Since protective levels of 3 vaccine doses develop by that time, you may consider yourself safe and free from rabies virus in your body.

Does rabies vaccine not work in preventing rabies with a person having low immune system?

It does but may be little less and therefore one more extra dose of vaccine may be given (5th on day 28 or even 6th on day 90).

In such scenario, blood levels of antibodies are the perfect guide.

Immunoglobulin given in the beginning will work even when host immunity is low and becomes important part of the treatment plan for this very reason.

Since there is no alternative to vaccine, it has to be given, even if lesser response is expected.

Can you get rabies twice? Why/ why not?

One may have exposure to rabies infection multiple times but immunization in time can save him.

If someone develops rabies disease, this is one time and last time affair.

What are the chances of my 45-day-old lab puppy having rabies? He does not play with other dogs and his mother was vaccinated.

Since there is no source of infection, your puppy seems safe.

Can I take a booster of rabies vaccine after 22 years of 3 doses of PrEP course? Will the antibodies still have memory in my blood?

Once vaccinated, immune system develops the know-how of making those particular antibodies and these remain in system memory for long time, probably life time. It was found that two booster doses brought immune levels high even when immune titers were not detectable before that in a previously immunized person.

Any booster dose will restart that factory and antibody formation starts.

Do I need anti-rabies after an eagle scratch?

Eagle being a bird, as such can't spread rabies; still there is remote possibility of rabies through eagle.

Eagle being a meat eater, if by chance carries rabies virus on its beak or claws after eating meat of rabid animal may transmit virus by scratch.

Once you have washed clean that scratch, most if not all of the virus if present is removed.

Chance of suffering rabies is rare but theoretically possible.

Better to take ARV to be 100% safe.

Could a parrot's bite cause rabies?

No. Only mammals can spread rabies and not birds.

A dog bit me today, but there was no skin puncture or scratch. Do I still need a vaccination?

No. Thorough cleaning should be enough.

Can Rabies Be Transmitted to Humans By Consuming Milk From Infected Cow or Buffalo?

Theoretically, there can be some risk when milk is used raw and there is some cut or wound in mouth till stomach.

When such milk reaches stomach, acid in stomach kills virus.

Boiling or pasteurization of milk will kill the entire virus load and that is why it is always advisable.

So far, no case is on record, who developed rabies because of drinking milk of a suspected rabid animal.

What is the best option when going to India if there's not enough time to get the rabies vaccination?

1. Best is to start immunization as per the protocol for "**pre-exposure prophylaxis**". It means you have to take total 2 doses of vaccine at day 0 and 7. Start it now and schedule may be completed in India. If you have taken anti rabies vaccine in past, two booster doses on day 0 and 3 will suffice.

2. Keep away from street dogs and un-immunized pet dogs as far as possible.

Thank you for your answer. Do Indian vaccines tend to have the same composition as found in Europe?

Yes, the same composition, best quality and much economical.

I am going to Thailand to work with elephants. Do I need to have rabies vaccination?

Yes you should.

Although elephants are less likely to have rabies, all warm blooded animals may be carriers or sufferers. Moreover anyone working in forests is likely to have risk of contact with other animals too. Vaccine availability at remote places may also be an issue. Third issue is cost.

Why not to be prepared in advance?

You need to take 2 doses, on day 0 and 7. This will be your pre-exposure prophylaxis.

Do people with potential rabies exposure need to be quarantined during post-exposure prophylactic treatment? If so, for how long?

No need to be quarantined as person has not yet developed rabies.

If the rabies virus travels through nerves, doesn't that mean the antibodies from rabies vaccine can't fight rabies since antibodies are blood-bound and nerves probably have no blood supply?

I'm uncertain if there is a direct answer. Indirectly, we may presume that immunoglobulin given/antibodies produced do reach nerves through blood supply and have their effect.

Blood vessels do not reach all brain tissue. Antibodies can not protect when virus has reached the target cells of brain and began making changes.

Although, I do not know if there is a clear answer, yet, **there is enough experience that no one dies when vaccine doses are complete before the onset of symptoms.**

[*Here are some supporting details, if you need:*

1. After inoculation, rabies virus replicate slowly and at low levels in muscle tissue or skin. **This slow initial step, likely accounts for disease's long incubation period.** Virus then enters the peripheral motor nerves. Once in the nerve, the virus travels by fast axonal transport, crossing synapses roughly every 12 hours. Probably when it enters the spinal cord it replicates and ascends rapidly to brain. Rapid dissemination occurs throughout the brain and spinal cord before symptoms appear. There are animal studies which have supported this point.

2. *Sufficient virus-neutralizing antibody in the central nerve system improves the survival of rabid rats.*

3. Medically: "A promising linear peptide of 29 amino acid structure derived from rabies glycoprotein is used to enable the entrance of rabies virus neutralizing single-chain antibody (ScFv) cross the blood brain barrier (BBB). This peptide has the ability to interact with the nicotinic acetylcholine receptors (nAchR) which enables the entrance of the antibodies in the muscle and nerve cells. *"Advances in rabies prophylaxis and treatment with emphasis on immunoresponse mechanisms".*

4. We all know that oxygen is blood bound but it reaches to every organ, of course via blood supply. Nerves do have their blood supply.

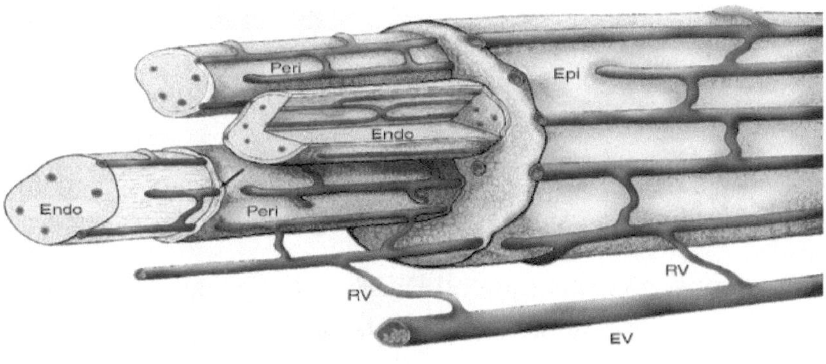

What is the vasa nervorum? It is the overarching term for the arteries that supply blood to the interior and exterior elements of peripheral nerves.]

Sir I have taken 4 doses of rabies vaccine after 3 years of exposure. As I have read that antibodies can't cross BBB. So is it possible that rabies virus remain dormant in brain and break out after few years?

Rabies virus may remain dormant in muscle tissue or progress towards brain very slow but once in brain, it works fast. Dormant state in brain is not documented.

Since you are safe so far and 4 doses of vaccine are complete, you are out of risk.

Enjoy life and thank nature that did not punish you for 3 years delay.

Or may be, there was no rabies at all.

When will a human become a carrier of rabies?

Human who has rabies virus in his body that has not reached his brain is in ' incubation period'. He will not spread virus in this stage.

When virus reaches his brain and rabies develops, he becomes a 'sufferer'. Soon virus reaches his salivary glands and secreted in saliva. Now he can infect others through saliva. In this condition, that person is in bad state and everyone will take care to not come in contact. This stage does not last longer and that person dies within few days.

Thus, truly speaking, there is no carrier state in rabies in humans.

Can pre-exposure prophylaxis of rabies protect if the rabies encounter goes unnoticed?

Yes it protects as our immune system notices the entry of any foreign antigen in the body even when we failed to notice.

This is the reason to recommend PrEP to those who can't report e.g. Unconscious, paralysed or mentally retarded, young children living in vicinity of animals or bat infested regions.

Can Rabies virus directly reach the brain through the olfactory nerves if the saliva of an rabid animal gets into your nose? Are ARVs effective in these kind of transmissions?

ARV is effective in Rabies in all the situations but problem is the time taken to be effective in first time user.

If that person has taken pre exposure prophylaxis, ARV only will be enough as it will show effect within hours.

This situation demands Rabies Immunoglobulin or even better Monoclonal antibodies for immediate protection.

Is it necessary to complete a rabies vaccination course?

No. It is not even necessary to start if it is not indicated.

Yes, once it is indicated. Rabies is not something to play tricks with it or take chances. Once it progresses, no amount of drugs and money can save life.

Complete the course once you start because it makes difference between life and death.

Why Not Vaccinate Dogs Instead of People?

Vaccination of humans after a bite is necessary, but expensive and puts a drain on medical resources.

Preventive vaccination of large populations of people is not feasible in terms of expense, discomfort, logistics and the small risk associated with vaccine.

But experts have shown that annual vaccinations of dogs can eliminate canine rabies, thus stopping almost all human rabies cases. Dog vaccination has eliminated rabies as a major public health problem in numerous countries.

I take only ARV shots. I missed the PEP dose. What do I do now?

PEP is 4 ARV shots only +/- Immunoglobulin.

Do not get confused with technical terms. Ask the treating doctor if any confusion.

My dog bites me many times and she is not vaccinated can I get rabies from my dog?

We believe in taking chances. we believe in taking risk.

We do not believe the literature, we do not believe in news and we hardly take any advice seriously, more so when it is health related.

Taking risk with something that is known to be 100% lethal may be your choice but is not the right choice.

Keeping a dog as pet that is not immunized is a risky affair. In America this is an offence and is punishable by law.

Pet and owner both un-immunized is a deadly combination.

Please take vaccine for both. There is no excuse.

CHAPTER 04

Why so Much Confusion with Rabies Vaccine and its Schedule?

This is the issue for both, the sufferers as well as health care providers.

People are confused with technical terms, with dates of scheduling and how to manage if scheduled date is missed.

When booster doses are needed, is another most asked question.

Confusion arise because Rabies has variable incubation period in both animals as well as in humans. Because of this, the vaccine is given even when patient reaches late, giving wrong notion that late vaccination is also okay. People start searching alternative option causing delay in vaccination.

Let us first take a look at WHO recommended schedule.

Rabies vaccines and immunoglobulins: WHO position April 2018

The April 2018 position paper replaces the 2010 WHO position on rabies vaccines. It presents new evidence in the field of rabies and the use of rabies vaccines, focusing on programmatic feasibility, simplification of vaccination schedules and improved cost- effectiveness.

The recommendations concern the two main immunization strategies, namely vaccination for post-exposure prophylaxis (PEP) and vaccination for pre-exposure prophylaxis (PrEP). The following sections summarize the main points of the updated WHO position as endorsed by the Strategic Advisory Group of Experts on immunization (SAGE) at its meeting in October 2017. [1]

Background

Rabies is a viral zoonotic disease responsible for an estimated 59,000 human deaths and over 3.7 million disability-adjusted life years (DALYs) lost every year.2 Rabies is almost invariably fatal once clinical signs occur, as a result of acute progressive encephalitis. Rabies occurs mainly in underserved populations, both rural and urban.3 Most cases occur in Africa and Asia, with approximately 40% of cases in children aged <15 years.

Mass vaccination campaigns targeting dogs is the principal strategy for rabies control by interrupting rabies virus (RABV) transmission between dogs and reducing transmission to humans and other mammals. Human-to-human transmission of rabies has never been confirmed, except extremely rarely as a result of infected tissue and organ transplantation.4,5

The primary diagnosis of rabies relies on clinical presentation and history of exposure to a suspect rabid animal or RABV.

Rabies vaccines can be administered by two different routes, intradermal (ID) or intramuscular (IM), and according to different schedules.

WHO Position: Administration of rabies vaccines:

[World Health Organization. Rabies vaccines: WHO Position Paper, April 2018 Recommendations. Vaccine. 2018;36:5500-3].

Route of administration: IM (Intra Muscular) or ID (Intra Dermal)

Site of administration:

- Intradermal (in skin) route: Deltoid region (shoulder), antero lateral(side portion) of thigh or supra scapular region
- Intramuscular (in muscle) route: Deltoid region and antero lateral thigh for age above 2 years.
- Only antero-lateral thigh for age below 2 years, avoid deltoid (shoulder)

- Rabies vaccine is not to be administered in gluteal area.

Volume of dose: One ID dose is 0.1 ml of vaccine and one IM dose is an entire vial of vaccine (0.5 ml or 1 ml in different brands).

WHO recommends **2 main immunization strategies for the prevention of human rabies:**

i. Pre-exposure prophylaxis (bebore bite) **(PrEP)**

ii. Post-exposure prophylaxis (after bite) **(PEP)**

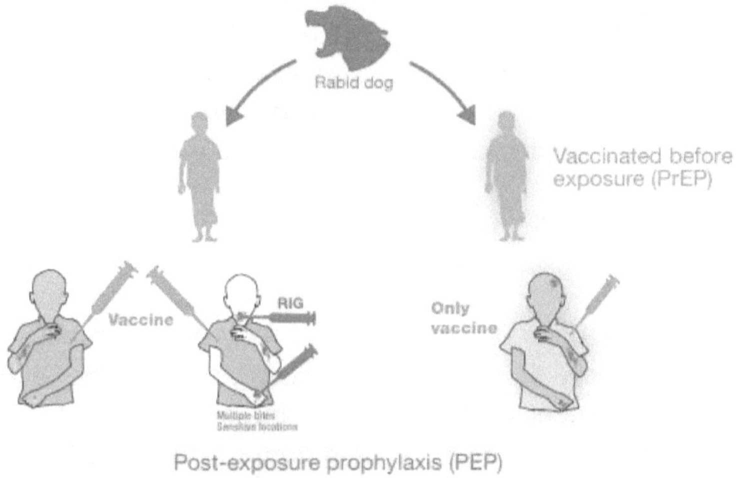

Pre-exposure prophylaxis (PrEP)

Pre-exposure prophylaxis (PrEP) is the administration of **two doses** of rabies vaccine before exposure to rabies virus.

PrEP is recommended for individuals at higher risk due to occupation. PrEP should be considered in sub-populations living in remote endemic areas (the dog bite incidence is >5% per year or vampire bat rabies is there), where access to PEP is difficult. Subsequent rabies vaccine boosters such as PEP when exposed, immunity can be recalled very effectively even decades after PrEP. To be precise if some one has received rabies vaccine in past it helps in quick respose when another dose is given, even after several years/decades.

For individuals (of any age) who have never received Rabies vaccine, WHO recommends the following PrEP schedules:

A 2 sites ID or a 1-site IM vaccine administration on **days 0 and 7 (Two doses in total).**

A routine PrEP booster or serology for neutralizing antibody titers (blood levels of protiene which kills rabies) recommended only if a continued, high risk of rabies exposure remains and in individuals with documented immunodeficiency (those who can not fight infection because of some defect in their immune system eg blood cancer, some medicine). They should be evaluated on a case-by-case basis and best receive an ID or IM PrEP schedule as above, plus a third vaccine administration between days 21 to 28. In them, additionally, in the event of an exposure, a complete PEP course, including RIG, is recommended.

Post-exposure prophylaxis (PEP)

PEP consists of the following steps:

1. All bite wounds, scratches and RABV-exposure sites should be attended to as soon as possible after the exposure; thorough washing and flushing of the wound for approximately 15 minutes, with soap or detergent and copious amounts of water, is required. Where available, an iodine-containing, or similarly viricidal (which kills virus), topical preparation should be applied to the wound.

2. A series of rabies vaccine injections should be administered promptly after an exposure.

3. **RIG should be administered for severe category III exposures**. Wounds that require suturing should be loosely sutured.

WHO recommends PEP for category II and III exposures. **The WHO rabies exposure categories are:**

Category I	touching or feeding animals, animal licks on intact skin (no exposure);

Category II nibbling of uncovered skin, minor scratches or abrasions without bleeding (exposure);

Category III single or multiple transdermal bites or scratches,

- contamination of mucous membrane or broken skin with saliva from animal lick,
- exposures due to direct contact with bats (severe exposure).

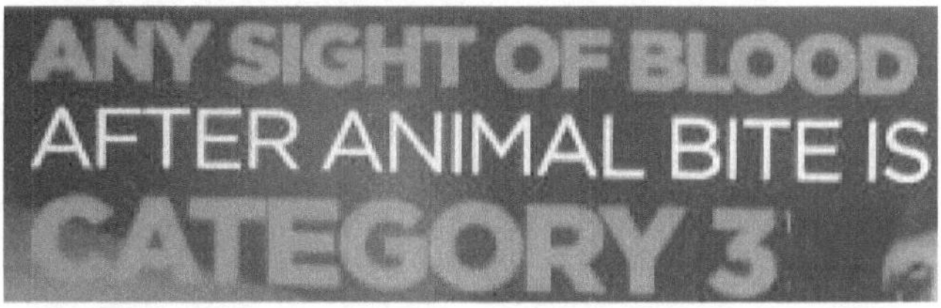

ID PEP schedules are cost- and dose-sparing and cost-effectiveness increases with numbers of patients seen in clinics.

If a repeat exposure occurs within 3 months of completion of PEP, only wound treatment is required, neither vaccine nor RIG is needed.

PEP recommendations by category of exposure

	Category I exposure	Category II exposure	Category III exposure
Immunologically naive individuals of all age groups	Wash exposed skin surfaces. No PEP required.	Wound washing and immediate vaccination: • 2-sites ID on days 0, 3 and 7 OR • 1-site IM on days 0, 3, 7 and between day 14-28 OR • 2-sites IM on days 0 and 1-site IM on days 7, 21 RIG is not indicated.	Wound washing and immediate vaccination • 2-sites ID on days 0, 3 and 7 OR • 1-site IM on days 0, 3, 7 and between day 14-28 OR • 2-sites IM on days 0 and 1- site IM on days 7, 21 **RIG administration is recommended**.
Previously immunized individuals of all age groups	Wash exposed skin surfaces No PEP required.	Wound washing and immediate vaccination*: • 1-site ID on days 0 and 3; OR • at 4-sites ID on day 0; OR • at 1-site IM on days 0 and 3; **RIG is not indicated**.	Wound washing and immediate vaccination*: • 1-site ID on days 0 and 3; OR • at 4-sites ID on day 0; OR • at 1-site IM on days 0 and 3; **RIG is not indicated**.

** except if complete PEP already received within <3 months previously*

Changes in rabies vaccine product and/or the route of administration during the same PEP course are acceptable, if unavoidable, to ensure PEP course completion.

Should a vaccine dose be delayed for any reason, the PEP schedule should be resumed (not restarted).

Individuals with documented immunodeficiency should be evaluated on a case-by-case basis and receive a complete course of ID or IM PEP, **including RIG**.

Rabies immunoglobulin administration

RIG provides passive immunization and is administered only once, as soon as possible after the initiation of PEP and not beyond day 7 after the first dose of vaccine. Correctly administered, RIG neutralizes the virus at the wound site within a few hours.

eRIG is less costly than hRIG, both have shown similar clinical outcomes in preventing rabies. As eRIG products are now highly purified, skin testing before administration is unnecessary and should be abandoned.

- Rabies Monoclonal antibodies can be used in dose of 3.33 IU/Kg-Rabiwax or 40IU/Kg- Twin rax in place of any RIG.

  To confer the maximum public health benefit, WHO recommends the following:

- The maximum dose is 20 IU (hRIG) and 40 IU (eRIG) per kg body weight. There is no minimum dose.

- Infiltrate as much as possible into the wound; the remainder of the calculated dose of RIG **does not need to be injected IM** at a distance from the wound **but can be fractionated in smaller, individual syringes to be used for other patients, aseptic retention given.**

If RIG is not available, thorough, prompt wound washing, together with immediate administration of the first vaccine dose, followed by a complete course of rabies vaccine, is highly effective in preventing rabies.

Vaccines should never be withheld, regardless of the availability of RIG.

If a limited amount of RIG is available, RIG allocation should be prioritized for exposed patients based on the following criteria: Multiple bites, deep wounds, bites to highly innervated parts of the body (such as head, neck and hands), severe immunodeficiency, the biting animal is a confirmed or probable rabies case, and bites, scratches or exposures of mucous membranes caused by a bat.

National Rabies Control Programme (of India)

National Guidelines on Rabies Prophylaxis revised after extensive expert consultations after newly endorsed WHO recommendations for Rabies prophylaxis in WHO TRS 1012.

NATIONAL CENTRE FOR DISEASE CONTROL (Directorate General of Health Services) 22-SHAM NATH MARG, DELHI - 110 054 hp://www.ncdc.gov.in 2015

Post-Exposure Prophylaxis (PEP)

ID route: Updated Thai Red Cross Schedule (2-2-2-0-2).

IM route: Essen regimen (1-1-1-1-1): Five dose intramuscular schedule - administration of five injections, one dose each given on days 0, 3, 7, 14 and 28.

Pre-exposure vaccination (PrEP): is administered as one full dose of vaccine IM or 0.1 ml ID on days 0, 7 and either day 21 or 28. (Total 3 doses)

Re-exposure in previously vaccinated person: only two booster doses IM or ID (0.1 ml at 1 site) on days 0 and 3.

Recent guidelines (2019) for Post-exp prophylaxis are available on NCDC website. These guidelines differ from WHO guidelines and recommend 5 doses for PEP and 3 for PrEP as earlier. All other recommendations remain the same. After extensive consultations with WHO, Indian Council of Medical Research (ICMR) needed sufficient data (of the studies that WHO had), to make the changes in schedule. That data is awaited.

Hope this confusion is resolved soon.

Till that time we are (medico-legally) bound to follow national guidelines, once patient is in India.

Health care provider has to face questions like many of the following because people can't understand technical jargon. Here are the answers I have been writing on Quora to explain them in a way that is simple to understand. Hope these are helpful to readers in day to day situations.

I was advised by a RMP (Quack) that one dose of vaccine is enough? Is that right? What is one shot for anti-rabies?

There is no single dose anti rabies vaccine for humans.

Those who are giving one dose only are badly mistaken.

One dose of vaccine does not porovide enough immunity required for full protection. In any condition you have to complete the course once.

I do not know how did this foolish idea propogated? Probably this is done by some ignorant people, sitting in position of authority.

This is why this book is needed.

Is one shot of rabies vaccine good enough for minor bites?

First, it's not the size of wound that decides rabies occurrence. Cause of rabies is a virus found in the saliva (of an infected animal) that has been inoculated by ANY type of penetrating bite into another animal/person's body. In fact, it doesn't even necessarily need an actual "bite". If a rabid animal's saliva contaminates ANY open wound or breech in skin, there is risk of exposure.

Regardless of size and site of wound or time of bite or type of clothes you wore you have to take vaccine.

If making a dish has 4 stages, can you make it in one stage when quantity is small?

Full immunity to rabies develops when 4–5 doses are given in a set sequence.

There is no guarantee of protection with one dose and if someone is doing this is misleading people.

Schedule is either full doses or none.

What is the difference between starting anti rabies vaccination on the first day and starting on the fourth day?

Difference may not mean anything or difference may be of life and death, depending on the severity of bite and incubation period in that case.

You must know that once Rabies sets in, there is no cure. Vaccine works when given before the disease is established. Incubation period varies widely, from 4 days to 3 years. Wound on head and neck or on hands are more risky as infection reaches brain faster.

So, why delay? Rush. Vaccine should be given as early as possible.

How many times can we take an anti-rabies vaccine in a lifetime?

There is no literature to answer this.

What is known is:

1. One full course of ARV gives immunity for more than a decade, may be 20 years. Although immune levels keep declining with time, immune memory remains intact even with undetectable levels.
2. Booster doses after any interval bring the immunity to its peak, that again will last similar duration.

Since this issue has not been researched extensively and as the disease is 100% lethal, we are advised to repeat boosters on every re-exposure (after 3 months). Although it seems contradictory to the existing knowledge (of longer immunity), no one must risk his life till final verdict comes from scientific community.

Since rabies is not the problem for advanced countries where most of the research takes place, no one is in hurry to establish an answer.

Till that time, keep taking the boosters on every re-exposure, whenever bite happens. At the same time, you should prevent yourself from repeat dog bites. Why should dogs bite you so often unless you are a vet?

Is it ok to get multiple rabies shots in a ten year period?

Maximum is one time full course and 2 boosters every 91 days thereafter, if needed.

Only question here is **'if needed'**. To save life it is essential even if there are any side effects, which really are not there.

Why do some countries recommend 4 doses and others 5 doses of rabies vaccine?

Earlier schedule was of 5 doses.

WHO, in 2018, after several studies on efficacy of modern vaccines has reduced it to a schedule of 4 doses, to be given on day 0, 3, 7, 14–28.

Some countries have adopted new schedule, rest are in the process.

On the similar lines pre exposure schedule now has only 2 doses instead of 3 on day 0 and 7.

Two Booster doses are recommended after every re-exposure whenever it happens after 90 days.

Ref: *World Health Organization. Rabies vaccines: WHO Position Paper, April 2018 Recommendations. Vaccine. 2018;36:5500-3.*

What if I take five doses of anti rabies vaccine in pre-exposure such as it is taken in post-exposure?

You get equal protection at higher cost.

When two doses can serve the same purpose, why wasting vaccine and your hard earned money?

No harm, otherwise.

What is the immunity duration between Pre exposure prophylaxis and post exposure prophylaxis? The vet said PEP has more immunity and permanent (because of 4 or 5 shots) than PrEP. Is that true?

No.

Vaccine is same.

Purpose of vaccination is same.

Only difference is in schedule and number of doses. In pre exposure prophylaxis, danger is not immediate, we are not in hurry and are planning for future but in post exposure we are under pressure to tackle the present crisis.

Effect is same and therefore duration of immunity developed is also the same.

I recently had a category 3 non-bite exposure from a stray dog. My last anti rabies booster was 5 years ago. Doctor told me that my immunity is no longer effective after 5 years & gave me the full PEP regimen (4shots+eRIG) is the eRIG bad for me if dog was not rabid?

1. eRIG is not bad even if dog was not rabid.

   But RIG was in fact not required in your case even if dog was rabid since you have received the vaccine in the past.

2. Only 2 doses of vaccine would have been enough.

3. Your exposure was not category III as there was no bite.

If rabies vaccine only grants immunity for a few years and rabies can incubate longer than that, how do you know that you won't still get rabies years after the vaccination?

Because Vaccine will kill the incubating virus also.

The immune system, once it has been put in action by a series of vaccinations, will eliminate the incubating viruses. Viruses may be hiding in some sanctuary in which they would escape notice from the unprepared immune system, but once the immune system gets cranked up, it digs them out of their sanctuaries and kills them.

Can I switch from ID to IM route of administration of vaccine, mid way?

Efficacy of vaccine will not change by changing the route of administration but why do it mid way?

Giving intra dermal injection is a bit tricky. All health professionals are not experienced enough to do it and all the hospitals are not authorized for this. All vaccine brands can not be given this way.

IM administration is easy and al the brands can be used this way.

Therefore make sure the person is well trained in giving vaccines, specially with ID route.

I took 2 anti rabies booster shots on day 0 and 7. Do I need to take one on day 21 also?

Two boosters are on day '0' and day '3' and that is all (except in case of immunocompromised person).

Can anyone take the 3rd rabies vaccination on the 8th day if he missed on the 7th day?

Yes.

Try not to delay next doses.

What will happen if I miss the last dose of rabies vaccine (ID route) but I take it after 4 days? My schedule was 0, 3, 7, and 28.

It gives almost the same effect once you have taken all the doses.

If my dog has had rabies shot and I get bit do I need a tetanus shot?

Tetanus and Rabies are two different diseases and you need protection from both. In your situation, Tetanus shot is definitely needed if you have not received it in last 10 years.

Should I repeat one dose of my rabies vaccine if it wasn't administered correctly?

Better do it.

Sir, a stray dog bites a previously immunized person, the person takes rabies (0 and 3) booster dose. If dog was not rabid at that time and after 75 days a rabid dog bites that person, so does the vaccine work on that bite too?

Yes that will work.

In fact it works even when both the times the dogs were rabid.

Dear sir, does rabies vaccine for 1 year 5 month old baby and 29 years adult person is same dose and same schedule? Doctor prescribed 5 ARV for baby and 5 ARV to adults.

Yes, dose and schedule remains the same for all age groups.

WHO latest schedule (2018) recommends 4 doses of vaccine instead of 5 as used to be earlier (except for immune-compromised who need 5 or 6 doses).

I have taken 14 anti rabies injection (5, 3, 3 and 3) in a year. Is there any side effect?

Question is not only of side effects but of WHY did you take so many doses of ARV?

It means you were bitten by dog every 3 months. Is it not some carelessness that exposes you to other risks in addition to Rabies only.

Every booster, you took 3 doses where 2 were enough. Why should you take excess doses? This also means that you did not consult some doctor.

Excess doses do not have any known side effect but your money was wasted. These doses could have saved the life of some more people.

Can you get harmed by too many rabies shots? I had to get 18 shots these last two years. Is my health in danger?

Before answering I would like to ask **why?**

Why are you getting exposed to rabies so frequently? Is it because of your profession or your behavior?

Did any doctor decide about your requirement of vaccine or you only are the decision maker?

In case you really can't avoid exposure to rabies so frequently, better get your antibody level tested. If it is proper, stop vaccine boosters.

Vaccine may not harm you (we do not know till now) but probably you are wasting something precious, the vaccine.

Can I take anti-rabies vaccine for no reason? I am not bitten by a dog or something but I want to take anti-rabies vaccine. Will it harm my body in any form?

Is it a good idea to get pre-exposure rabies vaccine or just wait for post exposure when needed?

Why the pre-exposure rabies vaccination isn't more widely offered to humans?

These 3 similar questions, therefore one answer.

In fact, this is the ideal situation to protect someone before the accident happens.

This will get immune system the capability to generate immunity against rabies and will protect the person for several years This is called 'pre-exposure Prophylaxis' (PrEP).

It is all the more important to remember that purpose of vaccination is prevention.

Why then pre exposure rabies vaccination was not always emphasized?

This is because:

Risk of rabies has been reduced to almost zero in many countries by

- Vaccinating all 'at-risk' people
- compulsorily vaccinating all pets
- Eliminating all street animals.

  Therefore vaccinating everyone as pre exposure is not cost-effective for them.

Problem is with countries like India, having high prevalence of rabies and high number of rabies deaths because:

- Our high risk population is more and is mostly unprotected
- All pets are not immunized
- street dogs and other animals are abundant
- Bite is at times not reported by children, unconscious, paralyzed or mentally retarded person
- Inadequate medical fecilities

Then why not?

Probably because:

- We follow western models for everything even when our conditions differ
- Rabies sufferers are mostly poor people and children, that does not make a vocal group
- It does not make political sense and is no political priority.

Pre-exposure prophylaxis is always preferable when:

- Risk of exposure to rabid animals is more frequent, e.g. Veterinarians, animal catchers, people working in zoo and even people having pet dog or cat (even when immunized), if one is a postman or a delivery boy or working in forest
- You are going to areas where rabies is prevalent
- You are in area where treatment may not be available whenever needed or will be very costly
- Children above the age of 3 when they start going to school

Pre-exposure vaccination has definite advantages:

- Less number of doses required and therefore lesser cost
- You are prepared to face eventuality
- You have immunity ready and therefore no need to receive immunoglobulin on rabies exposure.

We, in fact need pre-exposure prophylaxis. There may be better cost-benefit ratio in developing world.

Cost of vaccine is much lower in India as compared to west and we have abundant indigenous production. Our retail cost is Rs. 350 (less than $ 5) per dose. If used intra-dermal, cost per person will come down further.

Hope we think different, think rational and think of our local conditions.

Why is the rabies vaccination not given to young children as a routine when so many other vaccines are given?

Is it possible to include Rabies in regular immunization program for children?

Ideally it should be and many Pediatricians tried to convince the Government to modify their policy.

Rabies vaccine can safely be given with other childhood vaccines. In Vietnam, it was given along with dose 1, 2 and 3 of DTaP at 6, 10 and 14 week and was found efficacious and safe.

In fact, all health programs are based on cost-benefit analysis and this vaccination does not fit in this criteria.

However, in my opnion it should be kept in optional vaccines. Pediatrician can discuss with family and decide if the child fits in the critria given above.

Finally, you must know that biggest sufferers (number wise) of dog bite are children and which is one more reason to protect them while vaccinating them from several other non-lethal diseases.

Only countries with very low incidence of rabies can be exempted but not ours.

I want to take two boosters anti-rabies shots without any dog bite. Can it do any harm to me?

No harm.

It will boost your immunity, take it if you are in postion of risk which we have been discussing repeatedly in this book

At what age should the anti-rabies vaccine be given to people?

It is not in regular immunization schedule but can be given at any age, whenever needed.

Mostly, it is given post exposure. Ideal would be pre exposure, wherever risk of exposure is high.

After completing a course of antirabies vaccines as pre-exposure prophylaxis, when is a booster dose needed? Does PrEP provide sufficient antibodies without a booster dose for at least a year after vaccination?

Any schedule, Pre or Post exposure, does not need booster if there is no further exposure. Initial doses made body capable of responding whenever the need arises. Booster dose is only needed whenever there is exposure.

Can an anti rabies vaccine booster dose be taken 12 years after pre-exposure prophylaxis? Will the booster dose induce a rapid antibody response?

Yes.

Booster doses may be given any time after pre or post exposure course of ARV, whenever needed.

Longer interval does not matter.

Once immune system has know-how of making this antibody (immunological memory), it will immediately respond to boosters.

Is it harmful to repeat a PEP 5 dose rabies vaccine again after 5 years on an only daughter?

It will not harm but 5 doses are not really required as only 2 boosters can bring the same effect.

Who told you that those who have more children need less doses and only child needs more?

One patient is one person, whatever his/her number among siblings.

Where can I find relative literature regarding the new protocol of rabies vaccinations which states that revaccination is not required for three months?

In WHO guidelines for Rabies. 2018

A booster dose of rabies vaccine which is given as 6th dose on 90th day is missed and it is taken late by 8 days. Is it effective?

Yes, it is effective. In fact, persons with normal immunity do not really require it.

If 5 doses of ARV are recommended then why another (6th) one on day 60 or 90?

6th dose is not in routine protocol. Only people with suspected low immunity are advised this 6th dose. Latest WHO protocol recommends just 4 doses in PEP for normal persons, not even 5th.

Do I need HRIG again on a category 3 re-exposure (I was vaccinated with rabies vaccine completely without HRIG (as the bite was category 2) before?

Once you have received a full course of ARV in past, you will never require HRIG, whatever is the category of bite in future. So no HRIG now.

What's the point of pre exposure rabies shots if you need more after being bit? What would happen if you didn't get the post exposure shots after being infected?

You have 2 different questions in your question.

Answers are:

I. Advantages of Pre-exposure vaccination:

1. You have some pre-existing immunity if animal bites, and that means immediate protection available to some extent (important at places and times where/when medical help is not available)
2. Develop full immunity within hours of booster dose
3. Immunoglobulin is never required, whatever is the class of bite

II. What happens when one does not take post exposure vaccine after being infected?

What you get is Rabies, leading to death. Here again, if one has received PrEP but not PEP, may be saved with pre existing immunity, if that was enough.

I have taken rabies 4 vaccines 3 months ago, but not in proper way. I took 0, 3, 10, and 19. Will it protect me?

It will but immune levels may be little different.

How frequently should a person get the rabies vaccine if he feeds and remains in contact with stray dogs? Considering I have taken 5 dose of ARV already 5 years back.

There are no recommendations in this regard.

Equating your situation with persons working with animals (Vets and zoo workers) it seems safer in your case to go for boosters at 2 years interval or else, you can be tested every 2 years to find out how much immunity you still have by periodic titer (antibody levels) checks and get boosters as and when required.

The duration of protection varies, so regular titers are necessary to assess the need for a booster vaccination.

Although ACIP guidelines recommend that booster vaccination should be based on the results of the RFFIT, the test is not mandatory and some veterinarians may opt for the booster instead of the titer.

What are my chances of contracting rabies due to eye exposure and what should I do? I have started rabies vaccine 5 shots after 12 hours of the incident.

What do you mean by eye exposure to rabies?

Is there injury (in eye) and saliva of rabid dog going in to eye? Vaccine taken will protect you.

You should have taken RIG or Mrab also as this is considered category III bite.

I was scratched by a cat 15 days ago. I started anti-rabies vaccination on 4th day and the doctor said there's no need for immunoglobin since the wound is small and it's in hand. If I've finished 4 doses now, am I safe?

Yes, you are safe now after 4 doses of vaccine. But, remember that size of wound does not matter, depth matters. Bite on hand is more risky as hand is more near to brain.

If you are re-exposed to rabies more than once within 3 months of getting a full course of ARV, do you need booster shots?

No.

Does this also hold true for booster shots? That is re-exposed more than once within three months of taking two booster shots?

Yes.

You are fully protected for 90 days of primary vaccination as well as booster.

Can I get rabies if I had taken an anti-rabies vaccine 5 times in 3 years?

With vaccination at such short intervals, you must be having good levels of antibodies and thus well protected from Rabies.

But important is to save you from such frequent exposures.

Hope you are not immunocompromised (having diseases which hamper immunity, on anti-cancer drugs, or on steroids)

If any doubt, go to your doctor and get your blood levels tested.

If one got all four vaccine shots after a possible exposure to rabies (as scheduled & before the rabies symptoms appear), is he 100% safe from all previous exposures? Does it mean completing PEP either immediately or after a week's delay is the same?

Once you take rabies vaccine before the occurrence of symptoms, you are safe from all previous rabies exposures, present or past.

Delay of 7 days may become a reason of failure if wound is big/deep and on hands, face, neck or head.

Do not delay if possible. Risk is not small; it may cost life.

WHO states that if re-exposure occurs within 3 months of completion of PEP, no vaccine required. Should we count days from the first shot or last shot?

From last shot.

If a person gets a rabies vaccine booster before the completion of 3 months of his previous shots, does his immunity get extended for the next 3 months?

Yes.

I ate chyawanprash during my rabies vaccine course. Will it affect the efficacy of the rabies vaccines? Do I need to take my doses again?

My answer says NO for both.

Do I need to get rabies booster shots if I may have had an encounter with a bat between the fourth and fifth dose? I started a PEP rabies vaccine course and received the first three shots (Verorab) in Vietnam and the last two (Rabavert) in the US.

Boosters not needed.

Your course of 5 is enough to take care.

If you got bit by a bat in a cave, will you get rabies?

This is a situation of high risk.

Although bats in India are known to rarely carry rabies but who knows when & where?

Safe way is to get vaccinated.

My dog bit my child in the face. What should I do?

Dog bite on face is a serious issue and has to be given urgent attention. Hope you have already taken him to doctor after thoroughly cleaning the wound.

If your dog is vaccinated and your child too, minimum is two booster doses of ARV +/- one tetanus shot.

If dog is not vaccinated and child too, you need to give Immunoglobulin or better MRab urgently in and around the wound. Then start 4 dose series of ARV. Tetanus also if not received in last 10 years.

If dog is vaccinated but not your child, better follow all above steps.

If dog is unimmunized but your child is immunized, he needs 2 boosters of ARV +/- tetanus.

Having pre -exposure immunization for rabies is big advantage in such situation.

CHAPTER 05

Vaccines: The Real Game-Changer

Rabies is spread mostly by our oldest animal friend. For 15,000 years or more we have lived with dogs, loved them, written poetry and songs to them, and buried them alongside us.

The disease is described in texts from Greek and Roman antiquity, and in an ancient Ayurvedic text, the Sushruta Samhita. Some of the old records suggest an understanding that it was the saliva that transmitted the disease. But it wasn't until Pasteur developed it's vaccine more than a century ago that anything could be done.

Virtually all infections with rabies resulted in death until two French scientists, **Louis Pasteur and Émile Roux**, developed the first rabies vaccine in 1885. Nine-year-old **Joseph Meister** (1876–1940), who had been mauled by a rabid dog, was the first human to receive this vaccine. This was followed by an improved version of vaccine in 1908. Now we have much improved version for everyone in need.

Millions of people globally have been vaccinated so far and it is estimated that this saves more than 250,000 lives a year.

Rabies vaccine is on the World Health Organization's List of Essential Medicines, the safest and most effective medicines needed in a health system.

Available Vaccines

I. Cell Culture Vaccines (CCVs) include

- Purified chick embryo cell culture vaccine (PCECV)
- Human diploid cell vaccine (HDCV)
- Purified vero cell rabies vaccine

II. Purified duck embryo vaccine (PDEV).

[The human diploid cell rabies vaccine (H.D.C.V.) was started in 1967. Human diploid cell rabies vaccines are inactivated vaccines made using the attenuated (means destroying disease causing capacity of virus) Pitman-Moore L503 virus. Attenuated virus can still produce antibodies in host without making him sick

In addition to these developments, newer and less expensive purified chick embryo cell vaccines (CCEEV) and purified Vero cell rabies vaccines are now available and are recommended for use by the WHO. The purified Vero cell rabies vaccine uses the attenuated Wistar strain of the rabies virus, and uses the Vero cell line as its host. CCEEVs can be used in both pre and post exposure vaccinations. CCEEVs use inactivated rabies virus grown from either embryonated eggs or in cell cultures and are safe for use in humans and animals.

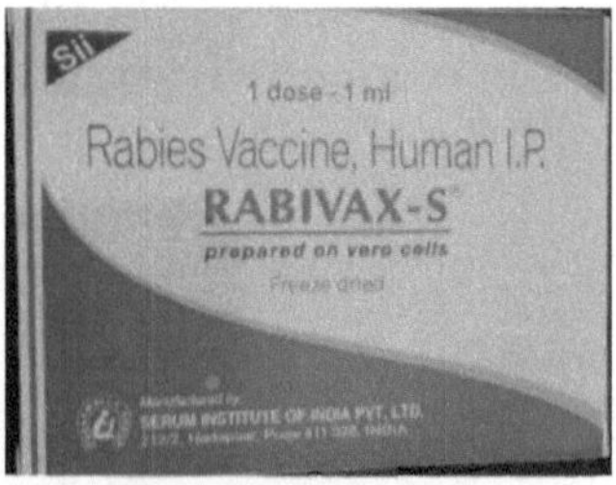

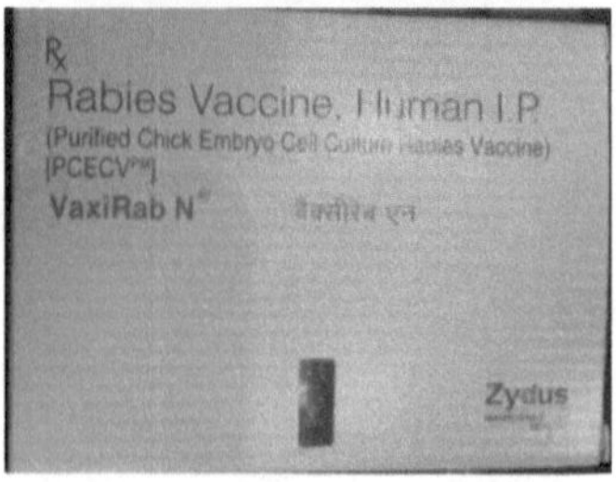

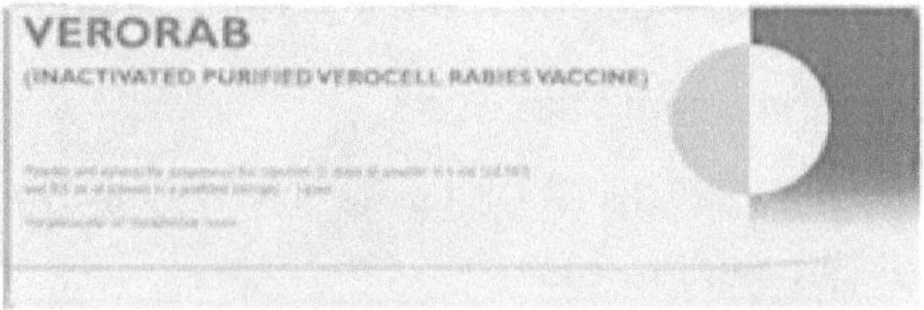

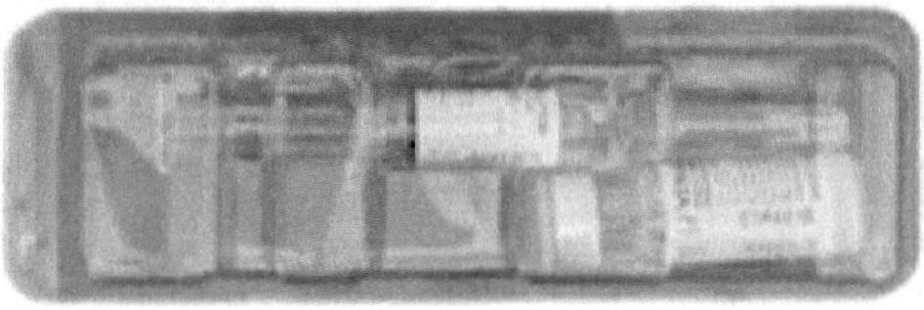

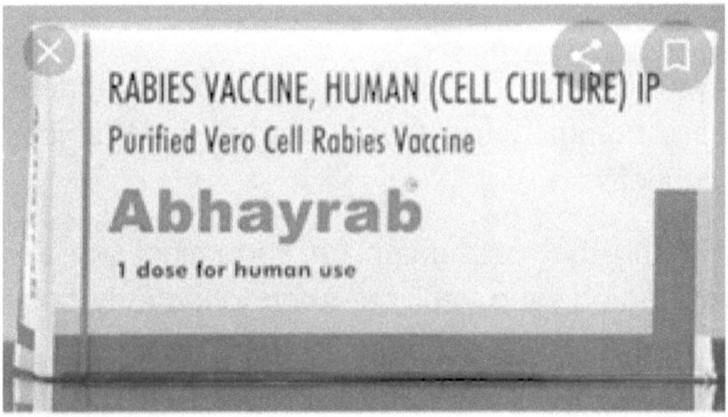

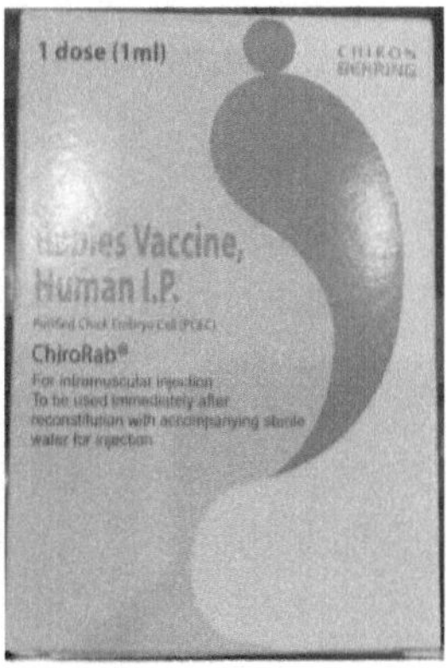

User need not to confuse with their details as all are made to confirm to same standards.

- None of these is given on abdominal wall as earlier nerve tissue vaccine.
- All are equally effective.
- Can be interchanged in emergency
- Same vaccine for Pre or Post exposure or booster schedule
- Same dose for all age groups
- High safety
- All indigenously made

- All economical, much by world standard, even free for poor
- Available throughout the world.
- These vaccines are available in lyophilized (dry) form to be diluted with sterile water.
- Stable for 3 years at 2-8 C and stable for 6 hours after reconstitution.
- They induce protective antibodies in more than 99% of vaccinees and effect lasts for 5-20 years. Booster doses give good (anamnestic) response even when serum levels were not detectable.
- Adverse effects are mainly local and minor like pain, redness and swelling. Less common are fever, headache, dizziness and gastrointestinal effects.

Large dose (7.5 ml or 15 ml) that was given on abdominal wall for 14 days is an old story of nerve tissue vaccine, abandoned long back (2004 in India).

Adverse Events after vaccination

CCVs are safe and well tolerated.

In 35–45% of vaccinated people minor, transient erythema, pain or swelling occurs at the site of injection.

in 5–15% of vaccinated people mild systemic adverse events: transient fever, headache, dizziness and gastrointestinal symptoms.

Serious adverse events are rare. Systemic hypersensitivity reactions may sometimes be seen with HDCV, mostly after boosters.

Fear and anxiety associated with vaccine: Q & As

Ignorance about vaccine is understandable but certain myths keep some people away from sure-shot safety.

Some people have suspicion that if vaccine is imperfectly designed, made or administered can itself cause rabies.

Some are afraid of injection, forgetting that death may be the result.

We face many such questions and yours may be one of them. Here are some examples:

Won't the rabies virus itself cause production of antibodies on infecting a person? If yes then what is the need of vaccine and Immunoglobulin?

On infection, virus can induce production of antibodies but it takes longer time. In case Virus produces disease faster, will kill the person before immunity can develop.

Are rabies vaccines safe for humans? Do they contain other viruses as they are cell based?

Yes, this vaccine is safe and does not contain any other virus.

Is it possible that in a hospital of human rabies, I was injected with a vaccine to cause the disease?

No. Not possible, not even as a tool of bio-terrorism, to kill one person at a time. A fool will do that. The person who administers such thing, surely be charged for murder..

There is no such injection so far to cause rabies.

It is your hypothetical fear.

Rabies kills few but phobia of Rabies or of injections makes many people sick.

Can rabies vaccine itself cause the disease sometime or strengthen the virus?

No. In no way can vaccine cause rabies.

This is the first question to be answered when any vaccine is invented and then permitted to be used.

This is the reason why human trials are conducted on thousands of people to assess the safety profile before it is allowed to be released

Think rational. These vaccines save about 250,000 people from rabies, year after year.

If someone takes an expired rabies vaccine, what will happen in his body?

Nothing.

Yes, I mean nothing wrong will happen because:

A vaccine is supposed to start losing efficacy after that date. It still remains the same vaccine but little less effective.

Practice is to not count that dose as given. Repeat it with new dose.

If you count this dose, it may give false sense of protection.

Is anti-rabies vaccination one of the predisposing factors for autoimmune diseases?

Never read about the connection of Rabies vaccine with autoimmune diseases but know that Rabies kills for sure and within days.

Autoimmune diseases, if at all happen will not be lethal.

Avoid seeking information from dubious sources.

Do you skin test the rabies vaccine?

That is not required. Even Immunoglobulins do not need be tested now as these are purified and safe.

I have been facing extreme amounts of anxiety and depression due to rabies, even though I have taken all my injections and booster doses 2 times within 5 months. How do you respond to someone who has become a Hypochondriac about rabies?

Think rational.

When you have taken something that is 100% effective, in double the dose, you have no reason left to worry about the rabies.

Now forget it and lead normal life.

If you still can't control your negative thoughts, take help of a Psychiatrist. You can overcome this anxiety.

What is the treatment of a person suffering from phobia of rabies and irrational fear of dog bite?

If somebody develops serious phobia hampering day to day life, it should be taken seriously and professional help should be taken.

Till then I am giving you some advice to explain to the patient:

- All the dogs are not rabid and every dog bite does not endanger our life.
- Rabies can never occur without saliva of rabid dog reaching inside our body.
- If vaccination has been carried out as per protocol, it is 100% effective. If efficacy is in doubt due to any reason, antibody level can be tested.
- If vaccination is delayed due to some reason but completed before the signs of disease, no one has been reported to die of rabies. This experience also means that disease can be averted by vaccine and Immunoglobulin anytime before virus has reached brain cells.

  No case of rabies has been documented in a person receiving the recommended schedule of PEP, since the introduction of modern cellular vaccines in 1970s.
- Very long incubation period of rabies is in very small number of cases. Most have the disease within first 6 months, major number in first 3 months only.
- A vaccine would not cause rabies. The vaccines are made with killed rabies viruses, so they cannot reproduce and cause infection. They are given to help your immune system fight the virus if it encounters it again in a live form.

If still not satisfied/confused/afraid, taking help of Psychiatrist is advisable.

In a recent rabies vaccine manufacturing scandal in China, authorities found that active ingredients produced at different times were used to make the final product. Some of the batches used were expired. What will be the harmful effects?

Biggest harm is putting innocent people's life in danger. All the persone received vaccine from those batches should be recalled and their antibody levels should be checked. The offending compony should bear the expenses of testing and revaccination.

Other harm done is the loss of credibility of the company and that company if proven guilty is likely to end in closure.

Since rabies is a 100% lethal disease once it happens and since rabies vaccines are considered 100% effective in preventing disease, and there is no treatment available for rabies**, assurance of vaccine with full efficacy** becomes all the more important.

False sense of protection given by this vaccine is unpardonable by any standards.

By and large, this incidence will harm the whole vaccine industry of China.

In India, we have 5 companies making this vaccine in sufficient quantity (rather surplus for export) and we do not need Chinese anti-rabies vaccine at all.

Does Dart tablet affect the efficacy of vaccine?

Dart does not.

What is the effect of Chloroquine when Rabies vaccine is being administered?

Chloroquine when given during rabies immunization with human diploid cell vaccine **intra-dermal**, may reduce its efficacy. It does not happen when same vaccine is being given IM.

A month old rabid puppy bitten me and died next day, I got rabies vaccination after 2 days, but now I am suffering from muscle spasm, appetite loss and joint pain, will I get rabies?

No, you will not.

Completing the full course of vaccine methodically, before the onset of symptoms of rabies, is the guarantee of safety.

Does anti-rabies vaccine have any side effect or is it safe to use? I was told by a government doctor that it is dangerous to use twice or more times after being bitten. I am so scared now and always living in fear. Should I take the vaccine or not?

These vaccines are very safe.

Use according to need. As such repeating also does not produce any different side effects.

What are the usual side effects of an HDCV booster? I had a full PEP series two years ago and have to get two boosters starting tomorrow. Terrified of ADEM/GBS.

When it is a matter if choosing between 100% fatal Rabies and rare possibility of neurologic disorder, I think choosing one is not difficult.

Moreover, rabies vaccines are quite safe and incidence of side effects is very low.

Can a person who is exposed to rabies and is taking rabies vaccine, transmit rabies to other persons?

No, not until the person exposed develops rabies himself. Once vaccination starts, chances of suffering are very slim.

If it is confirmed that animal/person exposed to rabies, can transmit the disease through body fluids if care takers have open wound or breech in skin, we must keep safe distance from the victim to avoid I infection.

Intact skin does not present a risk of contracting the virus if washed properly.

Why were the earlier rabies vaccines so painful and administered in the abdomen?

Earlier vaccine was different, less effective and with lot of side effects. That was 'nerve tissue vaccine'. Volume per dose was big, 7.5 ml-15 ml and therefore needed bigger area to inject. Every injection was painful.

Abdominal surface is the biggest area. 14 injections were needed. It saved from rabies death but process of immunization was really painful and scary. That was the only remedy in that era.

Present vaccine is much safer, more effective, is available in 0.5 ml or 1 ml volume and therefore can be given easily in arm or thigh muscle. Course is spread out over 28 days.

Has the rabies vaccine ever caused rabies (since they are dead viruses but could mistakenly be left alive?

NO.

No chance of mistake is allowed when making such vaccine.

Does taking Iodex Ayurvedic balm during my two rabies booster doses for headache affect the efficacy of rabies vaccine?

It will not affect the efficacy of vaccine. You may even take Paracetamol.

Can direct sunlight on an ampoule and a vial of rabies vaccine during reconstitution decrease its efficacy?

Although not desirable but it may happen sometime.

Effect depends on intensity and duration of exposure. Since it is not advisable to do so, we do not find any studies to give you exact answer.

Reconstitution of vaccine takes hardly a minute or two and this is too short a duration to have any remarkable effect.

Why is there a pain and tingling feeling at the vaccine area after 4 weeks of rabies vaccine? Is that a sign of rabies?

This is not a sign of rabies. It may be local tissue reaction.

Can I live a normal life, i.e. using household things, eating food, and drinking water with the same glass as others, while I am receiving anti-rabies vaccines?

After a bite, virus proliferate at the site of bite for few days and then moves towards nerve endings. It is not circulating throughout body. In nerves, it progresses towards brain through spinal cord.

When you receive the vaccine and antibodies form (or are given as RIG), will kill all the existing virus unless it has reached the brain.

In such situation, one is not spreading virus to others in any way and therefore can lead a normal life.

Secondly, all dogs that bite are not rabid. Many a times, vaccine is given out of fear, as we do not have any method to test and do not want to take any risk.

Is the rabies vaccine dangerous for a person with seizures?

No. There is no mention of any seizure related side effects of this vaccine in the literature.

Moreover, we have to outweigh between life and death.

Do all the anti-rabies vaccine doses for humans the same, meaning, the 1st dose is similar with 2nd?

Yes. Not only all 5 doses but even boosters are the same vaccine in same quantity.

Why should we give an anti-rabies injection around the wound?

This is not for vaccine but for immunoglobulin/monoclonal antibodies (ready made antibody to fight with virus before vaccine starts working).

This is done to neutralize the rabies virus at the site of entry only. If most of the virus can be prevented from reaching nerve endings, risk of rabies is reduced.

How does rabies vaccine protect, considering that nerve endings are located everywhere?

Vaccination against rabies (and against any other disease for that matter) teaches and trains the immune system to immediately respond to that particular threat, whenever that happens. This is like training the police force and keeping it in readiness to catch hold and eliminate that particular culprit, anywhere and everywhere in the system.

When a person is vaccinated against rabies he develops antibodies against rabies virus. As and when rabies virus enters the system, it gets recognized and neutralized immediately, before it can enter nerve endings, anywhere in the body.

At the same time we must not forget that risk of shorter incubation period is highest when bite is on hands or face as these are highly innervated areas. Such cases need prompt administration of Immunoglobulin and vaccine.

Hope this simplified explanation helps understand the mechanism of protection by means of vaccination.

Does a rabies vaccine protect you no matter where the virus entered from?

Yes, rabies vaccine once taken in proper dosage and schedule provides you immunity against rabies. All the tissues get this immunity. Virus is killed from wherever it enters the system.

How long does the rabies vaccine immunity last in humans?

And how many times in life can we take anti-rabies vaccine if needed?

There is no literature to answer this in clear terms.

What is known is:

1. One full course of ARV gives immunity for more than a decade may be 20 years although immune levels keep declining with time.

2. Booster dose anytime will bring the immunity to its peak that again will last similar duration.

This issue has not been researched extensively and as the disease is 100% lethal, we are advised to repeat boosters on every re-exposure (after 3 months) presuming that immunity must have declined somewhat. *Although it seems contradictory to the existing knowledge of immunity for long, no one must risk his life till final verdict comes from scientific community.*

Since rabies is not the problem for advanced countries where most of the research takes place, no one is in hurry to establish an answer.

Till that time, keep taking the boosters on every re-exposure. At the same time, you should device the ways to save yourself from repeat dog bites.

Another way is to check antibody titers (levels) every two years and act accordingly if your profession poses you at constant risk.

What happens if I take anti-rabies vaccine after having hydrophobia?

No use taking vaccine at that stage. Once disease has set in, vaccine can't reverse the process.

Is there a need to take an anti-rabies vaccine for a puppy bite if I'm still drinking an antibiotic?

Antibiotics are not anti-virals and definitely not anti- rabies. It is only the vaccine that can prevent rabies and no treatment available once disease sets in.

Think of ARV if other factors indicate.

If I take full rabies vaccination course after 1 year of dog bite? Will this work?

It works whenever you take it.

If you lock your door before thief reaches there, you are saved.

Issue is that one year is a long time of neglect. You are saved probably because the dog was not rabid. If you are in doubt due to circumstances, go for vaccination even now, because:

1. If at all rabies virus entered in your body which fortunately did not reach brain till now and produce disease, will be killed by this.

2. If you are not really infected, present course of vaccine will provide you immunity for future. This will work as pre exposure prophylaxis.

No harm either way, taking vaccine even this late is not a waste of money. This is investment in future.

Do My Family and I Need an Anti-Rabies Vaccination As Precaution Even When My Dogs Are Vaccinated Against Rabies?

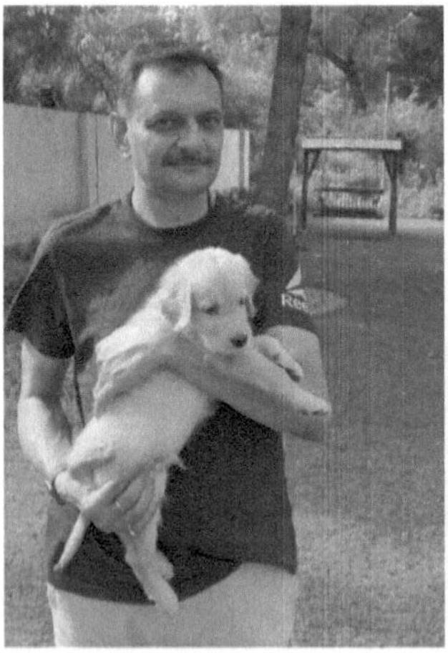

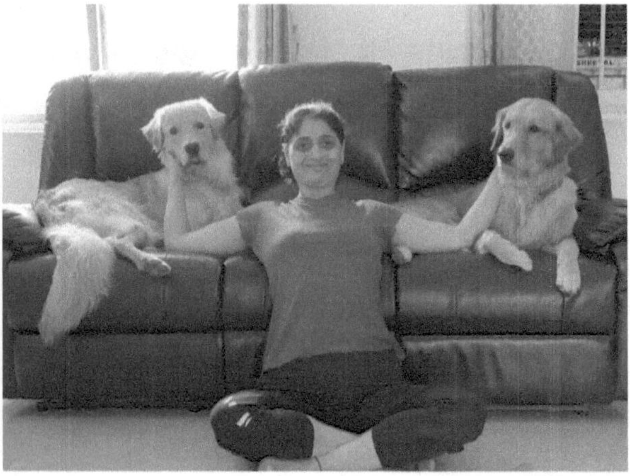

Yes.

That is the best strategy to get whole family pre exposure prophylaxis. It's once in life time affair.

Even when dog is vaccinated, we have no system of knowing its immune levels in case it's system did not respond well, or if vaccine was of lower efficacy.

There are several instances when pet dog scratches or licks and even bites sometimes, especially children.

If the rabies vaccine is given in the gluteus muscle is it completely ineffective?

It may be partially ineffective as absorption from fat tissue is not as good as from muscle tissue.

Can we take all anti-rabies injections in the buttocks?

In fact none.

You are not supposed to do it and if done by mistake, better not to count those doses.

Should I repeat 2 doses that I've already taken in gluteal region or taking the remaining three doses on

the deltoids would be enough?

As no one can give you assurance that first two doses would have worked well, better and safer will be to repeat. Remember that we need only 4 doses now for PEP (and not 5) as per latest WHO protocol

Does it matter if rabies vaccine are administered in alternate deltoid areas (left arm on day 0 and right arm on the 3rd day)?

No, it does not.

What if I take all my rabies vaccines subcutaneous?

It will not have desirable effect as this is not the recommended route of administering this vaccine.

Can I take 5 shots intradermal of rabies vaccine? After bite? 0 3 7 14 28

Yes, you can.

Even 4 doses are enough.

Points to be kept in mind when going for intradermal ARV:

1. It is given at designated centers where patient load is more and not in private set-ups where there is only one patient at a time.
2. Person administering must be expert in giving ID. Others may give it subcutaneous by mistake.
3. All vaccine brands are not used for ID route.

As an individual, you have no advantage in taking vaccine ID in place of IM.

The hospital will save on costs when many persons take ID in the same time slot.

Is there any possibility to develop rabies after the 3rd dose of ARV? Until now I am good and there are no symptoms, but could it occur now?

By the 3rd dose (day 7th), antibodies start showing in the blood means that your system becomes able to defend itself from rabies virus now. By day 10, reasonable amount of antibodies form. One who is safe till this time, should be safe thereafter.

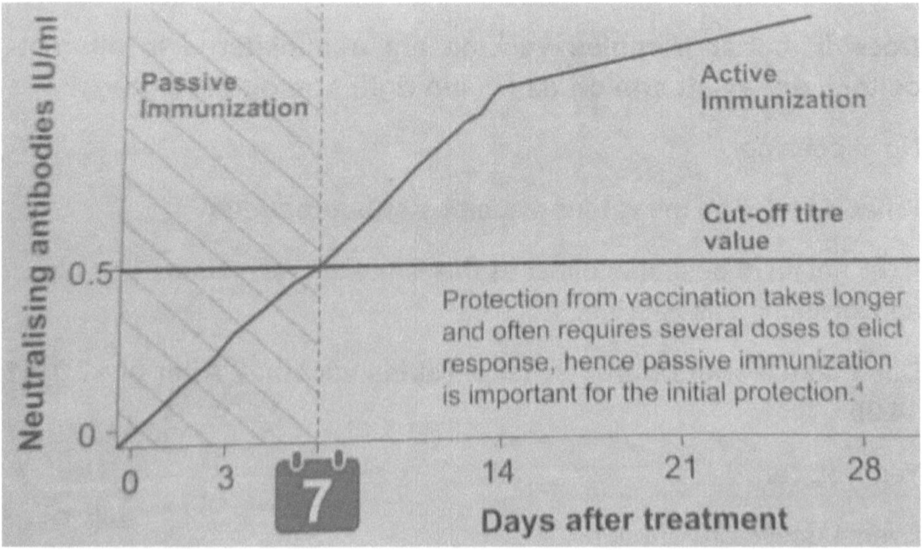

For a yearly immunized person, can PEP (4 injections), in which the 3rd dose was reconstituted in sunlight give protective immunity against rabies virus?

Yes.

Once a person is immunized yearly, has good immune level maintained. Two doses of booster would have been enough to boost his immunity to effective levels and he has received 4. Even if 1 of those 4 doses has little reduction in efficacy, it may not matter in end result. It does not mean that mistakes are acceptale.

Another issue is your yearly immunization with 4 doses, that is not really needed. Immunization (booster doses) is needed only when you have dog or animal bite.

If a person is bitten over paralyzed leg, would the vaccine reach everywhere in the body ?

Yes it will as paralysed part also has blood supply. Vaccine will kill the virus throughout the body.

What are the long-term side effects of rabies vaccine and how will it be?

No such side effects are reported.

Is taking an anti-rabies vaccine for the 3rd time bad? My doctor said I may become paralyzed in the future. I'm very scared.

No matter good or bad, that is not your choice. If it is really indicated, you have no options.

Doctor might have told you this probably because you may be taking vaccine without proper reasoning. Secondly, why should you need it multiple times; you must save yourself from dog bites.

In any case, taking vaccine for 3rd time does not cause paralysis.

Are all brands of anti-rabies vaccines effective like Rabipur?

Yes.

Which anti-rabies vaccine is more potent: Purified chick embryo cell vaccine or purified vero cell vaccine or purified duck embryo cell vaccine?

All these vaccine provide enough protection that is required for patient safety. All are equally safe. Cost is not much different.

Any one of these can be safely used.

When starting post-exposure rabies prophylaxis months later, are the same vaccines used?

Yes.

What is the cost of the rabies vaccination in India?

Vaccine About Rs. 350 per dose. (approx $ 5)

ERIG Rs. 625 for 5 ml of 1000U/ml (approx $ 9)

HRIG Rs. 5600 for 150 IU/ml, 300 IU vial (approx $ 80)

Human Monoclonal antibodies Rs. 2000 for 100 IU (approx $26)

Rs. 1000 for 50 IU

About the immune response, if one was attacked by a bat on the face & ear after receiving last rabies shot 15 days before; how long would it take for antibodies to reach the wound? Are there already antibodies everywhere in the bloodstream?

Message of entry of offending antigen to immune system is like calling 911.

As such, pre existing antibodies are everywhere. Our system escalates the production immediately so as to counter the offender as much as possible on entry point and nearby.

I know that Anti-Rabies vaccine is highly effective still can there be failure of prevention due to any reason?

Treatment failures or better to say failure of preventive strategy, if at all, happens rarely, one or more of following may be the causes:

- Delay in seeking treatment
- Improper wound care
- Unnoticed wounds
- Direct inoculation of the virus into nerve
- Lack of or improper administration of rabies immunoglobulin (failure to inject all bite sites)
- Vaccine failures: True vaccine failures are extremely rare
    - Lack of patient compliance with vaccination schedules
    - Improper cold chain
    - Use of vaccines that do not have their stated efficacy

CHAPTER 06

Rabies Immunoglobulins: Immediate Protector of Unprotected

It provides immediate protection to unvaccinated person.

These are of 3 types-

1. From animal serum (Equine Rabies Immuno globulin, ERIg): dose is 40 IU/Kg, max 3000 IU
2. From human serum (Human Rabies Immuno globulin, HRIg): dose is 20 IU/Kg, max 1500 IU
3. Genetically engineered (Monoclonal antibodies) (RMab): Dose is 3.33 units/Kg vial, 40 IU/ml.

   Twinrab: Dose is 40 units/kg

ERIg is economical. It is now available in highly purified form. This purified form can be given without skin sensitivity test

HRIg is very costly and not easily available since it has always to be imported.

Monoclonal Antibodies is the latest invention, best, safest and economical. Indian company is the first one to launch it in the world in 2018. It is easier to produce in bulk. All adverse reactions of blood products are avoided.

This is available throughout the country and is always preferable over two other alternatives.

The WHO rabies exposure categories are:

Category I	touching or feeding animals, animal licks on intact skin (no exposure);
Category II	nibbling of uncovered skin, minor scratches or abrasions without bleeding (exposure);
Category III	single or multiple transdermal bites or scratches, contamination of mucous membrane or broken skin with saliva from animal licks, exposures due to direct contact with bats (severe exposure).

Immunoglobulin is required in category III bites. It should also be given to immune-compromised patients with category II bites. Wounds that require suturing should be sutured loosely and only after RIG infiltration into the wound.

"WHO" mandates Active + Passive immunity **In Category III Bites**

Rabies immunoglobulin administration

RIG provides passive immunity with immediate effect and is administered only once, as soon as possible after the initiation of PEP and not beyond day 7 after the first dose of vaccine. Correctly administered, RIG neutralizes (blocks) the virus at the wound site within few hours. ERIG is less costly than HRIG; both have shown similar clinical outcomes in preventing rabies. As ERIG products are now highly purified, skin testing before administration is unnecessary and should be abandoned.

To confer maximum public health benefit, WHO recommends the following:

- The maximum dose is 20 IU (HRIG) or 40 IU (ERIG) per kg body weight. There is no minimum dose.

  Do not exceed the maximum dose.

In case of multiple wounds, the calculated volume of RIG should be diluted in sterile physiological saline to a volume sufficient to infiltrate all the wounds.

- Infiltrate as much as possible into the wound; the remainder of the calculated dose of RIG does not need to be injected IM at a distance from the wound (as was done in the past) but can be fractionated in smaller, individual syringes to be used for other patients.

  If RIG is not available, thorough, prompt wound washing, together with immediate administration of the first vaccine dose, followed by a complete course of rabies vaccine, is highly effective in preventing rabies. Vaccines should never be withheld, regardless of the availability of RIG.

If a limited amount of RIG is available (scarcity of RIG), RIG allocation should be prioritized for exposed patients based on the following criteria: Multiple bites, deep wounds, bites to highly innervated parts of the body (such as head, neck and hands), severe immunodeficiency, the biting animal is a confirmed or probable rabies case, and bites, scratches or exposures of mucous membranes caused by a bat.

Indian Journal of Medical Ethics CASE STUDY using a modified rabies immunoglobulin protocol in a crisis of unavailability: Ethical and practical challenges Omesh Kumar Bharti DOI: https://doi.org/10.20529/IJME.2019.022

[Abstract for your ready reference: Rabies is a dreaded disease of zoonotic (animal origin) origin, responsible for an estimated 55,000 deaths annually, of which 20,000 deaths are in India. Some animal bite patients need rabies immunoglobulin (RIG) for post exposure prophylaxis, in addition to the vaccine against rabies. The major reason for the high death rate in India is the high cost of RIG. Until 2017, the WHO-recommended protocol required a large amount of RIG. I describe how a cost-saving protocol for RIG was implemented in Himachal Pradesh. The published results contributed to the modification of the WHO's global recommendations on RIG use]

Dr. Omesh Kumar Bharati, received Padamshree for his this research.

ERIG administration

Although present day ERIG are highly purified, still Keep patient under observation for at least half–an–hour after ERIG administration as a precaution.

Following medicines should be kept ready — Inj.Hydrocortisone — Inj.Pheniramine maleate — IV Fluids, Oxygen — Inj.Adrenaline-1 in 1000, 1mg/ml (dose: Adults-0.5 ml; Children-0.01 ml/kg) — Deriphyllin, Dopamine, Ranitidine.

Administration of RIG/ Mrab in and around wound

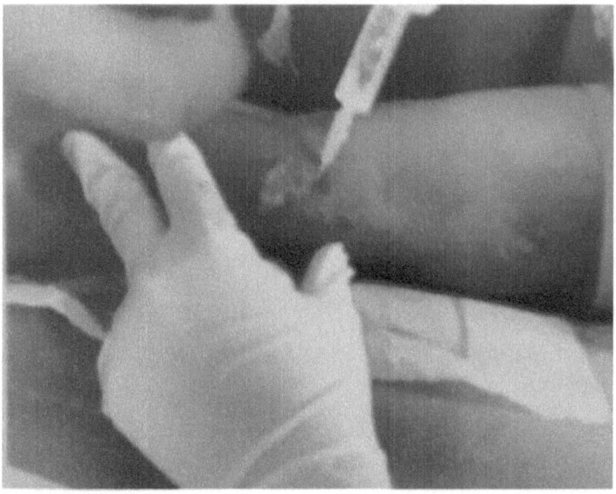

How to give so many injections to hemophilia patients with dog bite?

If dog bite is severe, there is no point in taking chances and Rabies Immunoglobulin has to be given for sure.

Since it needs to be given intra-muscular, surrounding the wound and may require multiple pricks, may induce prolonged bleeding when patient is hemophilic. Still it has to be given.

When wound is already bleeding and you are giving additional injections, you need to stop bleeding too. Administration of Factor concentrate is the best way to help. Local pressure on injection prick site for some time also helps.

For further course of 5 injections of anti rabies vaccine, spread out to 28 days, risk of bleeding is there but can be managed mostly by local pressure. Even better will be giving vaccine by intra-dermal route, that requires less volume (0.1 ml in place of 0.5 ml) and has much less chance of bleeding.

Why is Rabies Mortality in India High Even When All the Means of Protection are Available?

Other than ignorance and lack of medical facility in remote places, the major reason for the high death rate in India is not giving RIG to all who need it. High cost of RIG and non availability were supposed to be the reasons. Hope with the advent of Monoclonal antibody preparations, the scenario begins improving. Its availability can be insured and cost of management has also come down.

-WHO-	
35% of all patients requiring PEP Should receive both, the Vaccine as well as the Immunoglobulin.	Yet less than 1% receive that complete PEP (that is the Vaccine and the Immunoglobulin). This is the reason for many deaths.
Most important is initial immediate protection (by passive immunization-RIG) + Long lasting protection (by active immunization- Anti-rabies vaccine)	

Because of the cost involved, hardly 2–3% of the patients with severe bites received RIG (India and Thailand)]. Bigger reason I suppose is, no clarity of recommendations among heath workers and lack of political will.

With the availability of Monoclonal antibodies, this scenario is likely to change. Second change is accepting the Shimla (Himachal Pradesh) study by WHO in which using RIG leftover from other patients is permitted to be used for newer patients provided it is fractioned and kept in sterilized syringes.

Q & As on this topic on Quora that can make it's understanding better:

I was given 6 ml of equine rabies immunoglobulin just IM and not into the wound, can I get a second correctly administered dose 4 days later?

It would have been better if it was given in and around the wound.

But it will be safer not to repeat as equine product may produce adverse reaction when repeated.

If really indicated (ask the doctor again), go for Rabies monoclonal antibodies instead. This is safe and most effective.

What if an already vaccinated person takes immunoglobulin in a second severe dog bite?

Already vaccinated person needs two booster doses of vaccine and not immunoglobulin.

No harm if taken but no extra benefit either as antibodies might have been present already and are boosted as soon as you give one dose of vaccine.

But remember that immunocompromised persons have to repeat Immunoglobulin on every rabies exposure.

What if anyone does not take the RIG injection but complete the full course of ARV after a dog bite?

If dog is not rabid, no problem.

If dog is rabid and bite is in category III, you are at high risk till vaccine shows it's effect, that is initial 7-10 days.

I have taken 1st dose of ARV just after 3 hours of exposure. Now 3 doses are taken and one to go. At the day of incident doctors predicted the wound to be type 2. But after a week they doubted

by reviewing the wound that it can be type 3. But it was late to inject RIG at the wound site.

Taking full course of vaccine is enough if wound was not deep/big. After completing 3 doses you must have developed enough immunity. You cannot take RIG now (passed 7 days of first vaccine dose) and in fact you do not need it now.

For extra precaution, you may take 5th dose of ARV.

What are the maximum days by which anti-rabies serum can be given?

Begin vaccination and give dose of serum (immunoglobulin) as early as possible. All this must ideally begin at the day dog has bitten.

If for any reason immunoglobulin can't be given on day 1, it can be given till 7th day of beginning the vaccine. This can be *any interval from the day of dog bite*. As vaccine doses work and body begins producing own antibodies, ready-made immunity is no longer needed.

Why is it that healthcare workers want to give me HRIG shots along with boosters, when in fact I completed post exposure vaccination before?

Once you have received a course of anti rabies vaccine, whether pre or post exposure, your immune system has developed know-how of making antibodies at short notice.

In such scenario, if you have re-exposure, **you do not need HRIG**. Just 1–2 boosters are enough to raise antibody levels promptly (Unless you are an immunocompromised person).

You may ask them the reason of prescribing HRIG. They may be misinformed.

Can I take rabies immunoglobulin without anti rabies vaccine?

Yes you can.

But you must know that RIG gives protection for short time. If you are re-exposed, you are naive again and unprotected because RIG start dssapearing from blood within six weeks

Reason for taking both, RIG as well as vaccine together is that RIG protects you for the time being till long term immunity develops with vaccine.

Reasonable people think long term.

Does ERIg kill the rabies virus as soon as injected or does it take days to kill the virus?

Exact time taken by ERIG to kill the rabies virus is not defined but it must be in hours and not in days.

Is it OK to be injected with just ERIG instead of HRIG? I got bitten by my 1-month-old pup a week ago.

You have to take either of two. Please note that ERIG is RIG extracted from horse serum while HRIG is RIG from human serum. HRIG is more than 20 times costly than ERIG, not easily available but safer.

Now we have a better, safer and economical product for the same purpose, known as Rabies Monoclonal Antibodies. This is genetically engineered product, first time developed in India. (Find more details on page)

There are two important points of concern in your question:

1. Is ERIG equally effective as HRIG. Yes it is. Only difference is in the dose, cost and potential side effects.
2. Did you really require any of these? Probably not as your pup must have been at home and never exposed to rabies.

Taking ARV would have been enough.

Just observe your pup for any abnormal behavior and get the pup vaccinated at right time for future safety.

When will I be 100% safe after rabies vaccine taken 0-3-7 days but with no immunoglobulin? I have a stray cat's bite on the finger.

If you are normal by the time 3 doses of vaccine are complete (day 7), you are by and large safe as antibodies begin appering in blood. On day 10, antibodies are more and after 4th dose you can consider yourself 100% safe, even if you have not received immunoglobulin.

Does exposure to rabies on the ear or face (caused by a bat) always require RIG even when the person has completed PEP within a month?

Once a person has received a full course of rabies vaccine, pre or post exposure, has antibodies against rabies in his blood and therefore does not require RIG anytime in his life, wherever the bite is.

He only needs booster doses of vaccine on re-exposure after 3 months.

Can rabies immunoglobulin ERIg or RMab or (Rabishield) be administered in private hospitals?

Yes, it can be administered even in private clinic or in a rural health unit.

Since this is an emergency, assigning this duty to bigger hospitals only will make it difficult for masses.

Will the rabies vaccine work if rabies immunoglobulin is not given?

Yes but it takes some time, atleast 7 days to show reasonable effect.

Both are different but working for one purpose.

Vaccine is to develop active immunity while Immunoglobulin is ready made immunity (passive immunization). Immunoglobulin is to protect the patient till his own immunity develops by vaccine, that is first 7 days of vaccination. This is for first time user, who did not have previous immunity.

Two work sequentially in first time user.

What is new in Rabies management, an Indian product, that can change the whole scenario, for better?

This:

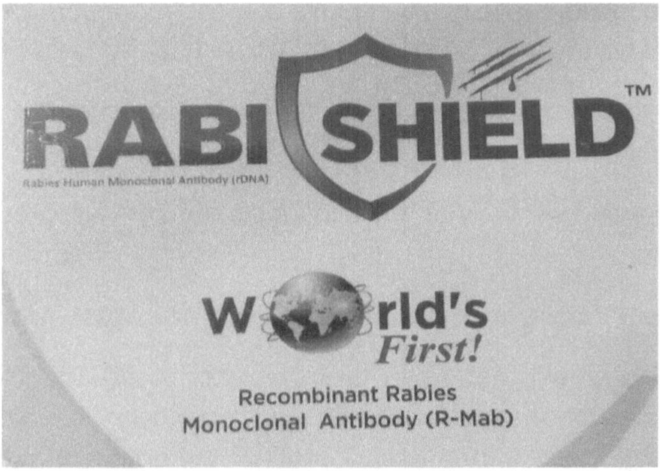

This is really something new, something novel, with proven efficacy and safest product in the class.

This is an product by an Indian vaccine maker, "Serum Institute of India" in collaboration with Mass Biologics of the University of Massachusetts Medical School, USA.

Like Rabies immunoglobulin, it provides readymade immunity against rabies till the vaccine develops immune levels. Mrab like RIG is therefore the first drug to be given with anti rabies vaccine in all severe dog bites (class III). Till now, we had two types of RIG available, ERIG and HRIG. HRIG had less chances of hypersensitivity than ERIG but is 20 times costlier and in short supply.

Because of the cost involved, hardly 2–3% of the patients with severe bites received RIG (India and Thailand). ***This is one of the reasons of high mortality from rabies.***

Because both RIGs are blood products, there was always potential risk of blood-borne diseases despite all precautionary measures.

Rabishield (Mrab) is a novel product that is not derived from blood. This is something genetically engineered. This is human monoclonal antibody against rabies glycoprotein by recombinant DNA technology on Chinese hamster ovary cells. (it is not made from human blood, it is prepared in lab to get rid of side effects of blood products). It neutralizes 25 different wild type or street type RABV isolates.

Presently, this is much economical than HRIG because of its smaller dose.

The whole world will welcome this invention and we are proud that this is from India.

This will herald the era of **'no blood based anti-rabies product'**.

Cost of Rabi-shield that was more than Rs. 10,000 per 100 IU vial at launch has been slashed by 80% within a month. This makes a revolution by making this safest product economical, equal to ERIG (dose wise).

PRESENTATION:

50 IU/1.25 ml vial Cost Rs. 1000
100 IU/2.5 ml vial Cost Rs. 2000
250 IU vial is not available now.

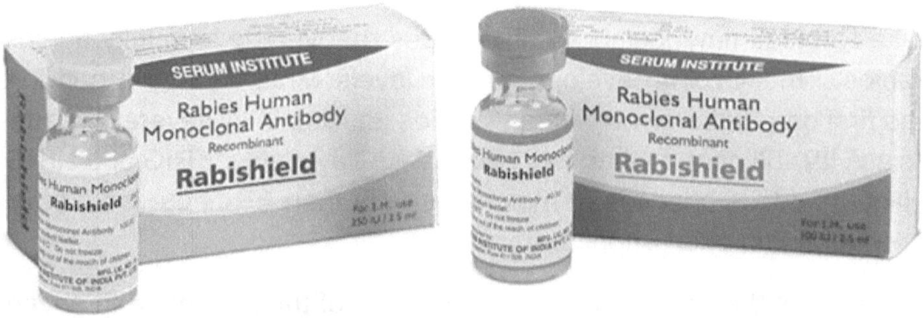

You may read further from following WHO document:

2018, 93, 201–220 **No 16**

World Health Organization

Organisation mondiale de la Santé

Weekly epidemiological record

Relevé épidémiologique hebdomadaire

20 APRIL 2018, 93th YEAR / 20 AVRIL 2018, 93e ANNÉE
No 16, 2018, 93, 201–220
http://www.who.int/wer

A single monoclonal antibody (mAb) product against rabies, which was licensed in India in 2017, has been demonstrated to be safe and effective in clinical trials. This mAb neutralizes a broad panel of globally prevalent RABV isolates. The comparative advantages of mAb products include large-scale production with standardized quality, greater effectiveness than RIG, elimination of the use of animals in the production process, and reduction in the risk of adverse events.

Anti-rabies monoclonal antibody from Zydus, TwinrabTM (RabiMabs), an alternative to Rabishield:

Zydus has received marketing authorization for TwinrabTM (RabiMabs) from the Drug Controller General of India. The novel biologic which will be marketed under the brand name, TwinrabTM, is indicated in combination with rabies vaccine for rabies post-exposure prophylaxis. The United States Food and Drug Administration (USFDA) has granted an orphan drug status to this candidate. In 2008, Zydus had entered into an agreement with the WHO to explore opportunities in the development of a **cocktail of monoclonal antibodies** for the treatment of rabies. The use of rabies monoclonal antibodies could emerge as an innovative therapy and form a potent alternative to current blood derived RIG. This product contains **two or more antibodies that bind to two different sites on the rabies virus**.

As TwinrabTM is cell culture derived, it offers high levels of purity including freedom from risk of infections as compared to the human serum derived products. TwinrabTM will be produced in bioreactors, making it easier to produce in large quantities.

Novel cocktail of two murine monoclonal antibodies produced by hybridomas Sourced from WHO partnering centers: CDC, Atlanta, USA and ADRI, Nepean, Canada - - M777-16-3 (IgG1) - Binds to site II on G protein of rabies virus envelope - 62-71-3 (IgG2b) - Binds to site III on G protein of rabies virus envelope. Risk mitigation: The binding of RabiMabs product to two distinct antigenic sites provides adequate protection against a mutated rabies virus that has lost an epitope due to a mutation.

Dose 40 IU/Kg.

Cost 1 ml (600 IU) Rs. 1697

1.5 ml (1500 IU) Rs. 3085

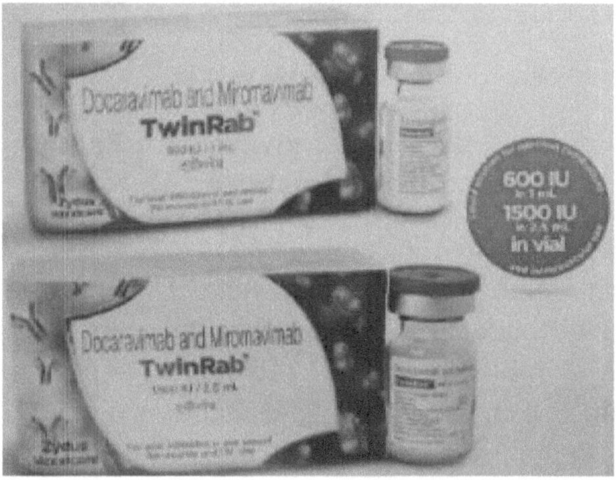

CHAPTER 07

How Do I Know That I Have Achieved Perfect Protection?

You do it by testing serum level of antibodies after giving vaccine.

This is an expensive test therefore not done routinely.

Not everyone needs to go for it.

The Rabies Titer Test or RFFIT (Rapid Focus Florescence Inhibition Test)

This is used to monitor rabies antibody levels in someone who may have an occupational risk of rabies, such as veterinarians or rabies lab workers, or someone who has been exposed to rabies and needs to be monitored to ensure that the vaccination is effective. Usually, testing is not necessary if the standard protocol is followed for the rabies vaccination after an animal bite.

Is antibody test easily doable? I was vaccinated 20 years back.

It is not available everywhere and is costly.

Centers in India estimating these titers are:

- NICD, Delhi
- CRI, Kasauli
- National Institute of Virology, Pune
- Pasteur Institute of India, Coonor, The Nilgris, Tamil Nadu.
- NIMHANS, Bangalore

In private sector, I have information about only PATHKIND doing it and charging Rs. 5600.

How Can I Stay Fully Protected Against Rabies At All Time?

I don't care about the cost. I am asking because bat exposure which can go unnoticed. Do I have to take vaccine every 3 month (will that hurt my immunity?) or blood titer test every now and then?

I agree with your concern.

Being protected against rabies for ever is neither so difficult nor so costly.

The way forward:

1. Take 2 doses of ARV at 7 days interval. This is primary immunization and is named "Pre-exposure prophylaxis". Your immune system now learns how to produce antibodies against rabies. You also develop a basal level of antibodies by this.
2. Whenever in future you are exposed to bat bite or animal bite, if it is beyond 90 days from last dose of vaccine, you have to take 2 booster doses at day 0 and 3. It will boost up the immunity to peak level again. Longer gap does not matter.
3. In case your profession is such that you will be re-exposed frequently, you may not take boosters like this, rather go for antibody titers every 2 years and 2 booster doses if titers found low (<0.5 IU/ml) (Ref: Laboratory rabies-laboratory/rffit-test).

Immunity by any dose of rabies immunization lasts beyond 10 years yet boosters are given to get highest possible titers at the point of need just in case it has gone down.

The day antibody titer estimation becomes affordable and available everywhere, need of boosters will reduce.

One more big advantage of Pre-exposure prophylaxis is that you will never need Rabies Immunoglobulin (RIG) or Human monoclonal antibodies whatever is the degree of exposure.

For these very reasons, there is demand to make rabies immunization a part of routine childhood immunization, in countries where rabies is prevalent.

When will I know that I won't get rabies after being bitten by a bat?

Once you start taking vaccine and by 3rd dose you begin having your own antibodies, you are in safe zone. By day 10 you have reasonable immunity.

How can I verify at home if I have rabies?

You can not even at hospital as there are no tests for it.

And when it is verified based on symptoms, it is point of no return.

If blood has a rabies antigen, what is its CBC report?

CBC report will show nothing specific that can help in diagnosis.

Can a bronze plate detect the presence of rabies bacteria after bitten by a dog?

1. Rabies is caused by a virus and not bacteria.
2. There is no test to detect the rabies infection till it is very late, even in animals.
3. There is no mention of the test you say anywhere in science literature.

My rabies antibody test is >4. Will I get rabies?

Rabies antibody titer above 0.5 is considered enough for protection and you have 8 times of that.

If the level 0.5 IU/ml is protective, can I rest assure that my completed series of vaccination is successful? (As no failure due to faulty vaccine from improper temperature, from steroid (high

doses) which cause immune suppressed OR whatever possible way that cause vaccination failure).

Yes.

Am I safe from rabies if antibody titer is 6.0 IU/ml after PEP vaccination of rabies which is taken after 2 months of a dog bite?

You must have been advised this test just to satisfy you.

You must have been given this report again with the good news that you are safe.

With antibodies 12 times the required protective level, you should not have any doubt being safe.

The RFFIT test was done after 4 months of vaccination and it was 32 IU/ml. What will happen if 4 injections of rabies will be taken after 9 months of the RFFIT test?

In 9 months, these immune levels will recede to some extent but will be boosted once you take vaccine, 4 doses.

Question is why will you take 4 doses again?

Once you are fully immunized and have such robust immunity, you do not need any boosting. Even then if you are taking, at the most you need 2 booster doses and not 4.

Do you know if a rabies booster shot will be needed for a 2nd exposure if my current titer is 4.5 IU/ML? I got my titer checked 8 days before 2nd exposure, can the titer change in 8 days or should I be in the clear?

Once you have such high titers, you do not need another booster at this stage.

If I take a rabies titer test 3 months after vaccination, and the result is way higher than 0.5 IU, then I do not need boosters for re-exposure for a while right?

Theoretically yes, you do not need booster at this point. This was the reason you went for testing.

Getting titers tested is a costly process and is not available to all at all the places while vaccine is.

After how much time should a blood titer test be done to confirm the production of rabies neutralizing antibodies in the immunized person?

Not advised and not done in normal persons. Still if considered, do after 7 days at least.

Does the rabies vaccine work within 7 days, or does it take more than 7 days to work?

Starts working from day 1 but protective levels develop by day 7 to 10.

Will nanotechnology really be used effectively to cure rabies or cancer soon?

This will definitely be a highly useful aid in the management of many diseases as and when it comes in to the realm of possibility.

It may help in target delivery of drugs.

In any disease, some particular tissue or cells are affected but whatever drug we give goes all throughout the body unnecessarily. It may have toxic effect on normal tissues (especially with chemotherapy).

If drug can be delivered to target tissue only, lesser dose will be effective and side effects will be minimized. Nano particles can do it.

Should I still be worried about rabies if a year goes after initial exposure?

Once you have taken vaccine in prescribed format, you are safe 100%.

If not, good news is that still there is chance of correcting your mistake.

Stregthening of Laboratory Diagnosis Of Rabies in India

India had only one laboratory for diagnosing rabies in animals, located in Bangalore at the Veterinary College of the Karnataka Veterinary, Animal and Fisheries Science University

Four regional laboratories have been supported under the programme to Strengthening Rabies Diagnostics

1. National Institute of Mental Health and Neurosciences (NIMHANS),
2. Disease Investigation Unit Lab, Directorate of Animal Husbandry and Veterinary Services, Government of Goa, Panaji, Goa,
3. AIIMS Jodhpur,
4. National Center for Disease Control (NCDC), Delhi)

CHAPTER

08

When Rabies is a 100% Fatal Disease and Dog is the Main Culprit, Why Do We Have Dogs at All?

When mosquitoes spread diseases that are curable, we apply all methods to kill them. When dogs spread a disease that has no cure, why do we tolerate them, domesticate them and even love them so much?

This question naturally comes to our mind when we study the deaths caused by Rabies. But when we look around, we feel that dogs are largely loved and existed with human beings for centuries.

Does it not mean that we must eliminate rabies but not dogs?

This makes interesting reading.

* * *

In 2018, an estimate of the global dog population was 900 million.

The human population at that time was nearly 7500 million.

It is said that the "dog is man's best friend" but this refers largely to almost 20% of dogs that live in developed countries. In the developing world, dogs are more commonly on streets or community-owned. Most of these dogs live their lives as scavengers, sometimes cared for by the community, however never been owned by anyone.

Having Pets is not merely an American phenomenon, although, in America, most people have a pet. Nearly 40% of American families own at least one dog. There are more pets than children in many families. Half of all dogs sleep in the same bed as a family member. About 90 % of pet owners consider their pets as members of the family.

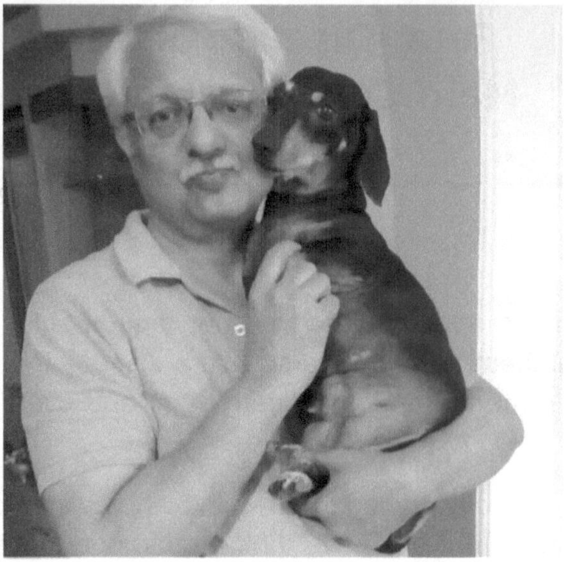

But they are very strict to save humans and animals from Rabies. Therefore, according to the ASPCA, approximately 2.7 million animals are euthanized at shelters (1.2 million dogs and 1.4 million cats) for various reasons and rabies is the most important.

In some European nations e.g. Switzerland, the pet over-population doesn't exist. The number of homeless animals is negligible. In India and many of the developing countries, most of the dogs live in the streets. Although most of the rabies cases in India are attributed to these dogs, culling is banned by law.

Also, the data offered demonstrates that just because pets are treated differently in other cultures, that doesn't mean they're not loved.

As a domesticated or semi-domesticated animal, the dog is nearly universal among human societies for centuries.

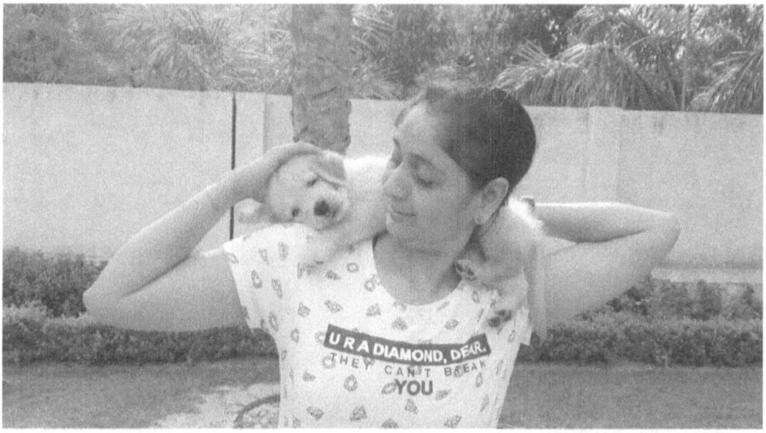

The dog was the first species to be domesticated and has been selectively bred over millennia. Their long association with humans has led dogs to be uniquely attuned to human behaviour and they are able to thrive on a starch-rich diet that is not natural for other canines.

They perform many roles for humans, such as hunting, herding, pulling loads and protection. They are being trained in assisting police and military searching narcotics, ammunition and land-mines. Dogs provide companions and, more recently, aiding disabled people and in therapeutic roles. Their powerful sense of smell may be used even for the diagnosis of certain illnesses. This influence on human society has given them the sobriquet of «man's best friend".

The minds of dogs inevitably have been shaped by millennia of contact with humans. As a result of this physical and social evolution, dogs, more than any other species, have acquired the ability to understand and communicate with humans. Behavioural scientists have uncovered a surprising set of social-cognitive abilities in domestic dog. These abilities are not possessed by the dog's closest canine relatives nor by other highly intelligent mammals such as great apes but rather parallel some of the social-cognitive skills of human children.

Dog is the most widely present terrestrial carnivore.

Domestic dogs inherited complex behaviours from their wolf ancestors. These sophisticated forms of social cognition and communication may account for their trainability, playfulness, and ability to fit into human households and social situations, and these attributes have given dogs a relationship with humans that has enabled them to become one of the most successful species on the planet today.

Reasons Why Dogs Make Good Pets

- They reciprocate your love and love unconditionally
- Instil happiness
- Provide companionship
- Provide security
- They keep you active
- Relieve stress
- Entertainment

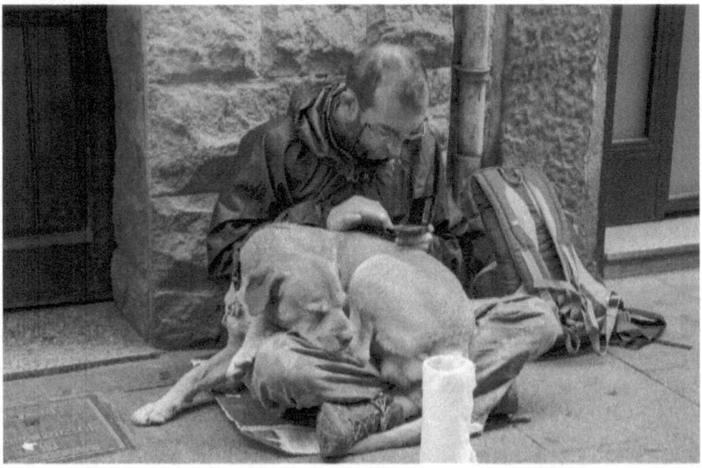

It would be great if we can vaccinate every dog that can come in contact with humans and their pets and possibly eliminate Rabies. Many countries have achieved this.

Was it not the only reason that we thought of killing all the dogs in this world?

Let us enjoy their companionship.

CHAPTER 09 Rabies in Dogs

Rabies is a fatal viral encephalitis that specifically affects the Gray matter of dog's brain and the central nervous system (CNS).

In the USA (except in Hawaii), it is legally required that every owned dog be vaccinated against the rabies virus. Such regulations do not exist in many developing countries.

Depending on local law, vaccination must be repeated every year to three years, depending on the rabies vaccine used.

Causes of Animal Rabies

The rabies virus is a single-stranded RNA virus of the genus *Lyssavirus*, in the family *Rhabdoviridae*. It is transmitted through the exchange of blood or saliva from an infected animal.

The primary way the rabies virus is transmitted to dogs and other animals is through a bite from another dog or wild animals like foxes, raccoons, skunks and bats that carry the disease. The virus is transmitted through biting and possibly scratching—it gets transferred in the saliva. Rabies is highly infectious.

Once the virus enters the dog's body, it replicates in the cells of the muscles and then spreads to the closest nerve fibres, including all peripheral, sensory and motor nerves, traveling from there to the brain. The virus usually takes less than 10 days to develop but at times it may take even a month. Once rabies symptoms have begun, the virus progresses rapidly.

Symptoms and Types of Rabies in Dogs

There are two forms of rabies among dogs: paralytic and furious. In the early (prodromal) stage of rabies infection, a dog will show only mild signs of CNS abnormalities. This stage will last from one to three days. Most dogs will then progress to either the furious stage or the paralytic stage, or a combination of the two, while others succumb to the infection without displaying any major symptoms. Furious rabies in dogs is characterized by extreme behavioural changes, including overt aggression and attack behaviour. Paralytic rabies, also referred to as dumb rabies, is characterized by weakness and loss of coordination, followed by paralysis.

This is a virus that acts fast. If it is not addressed before the symptoms of rabies have begun, the prognosis is grave. Therefore, if your dog has been with another animal, or has been bitten or scratched by another animal, or if you have any reason to suspect that your pet has come into contact with a rabid animal (even if your pet is vaccinated against rabies), you must take the dog to a veterinarian for preventive care immediately. Do not wait for symptoms, because by then it is too late to save the pet.

Diagnosing Rabies in Dogs

If your dog has received the vaccines in time, the veterinarian will give your pet a booster dose of the dog rabies vaccine and then quarantine him for 10 days. If your dog bit a human or is not up to date on his rabies vaccine, the next step will depend on state or local laws but usually includes mandatory quarantine. Rabies can be confused with other conditions that cause aggressive behaviour, so a diagnosis is based on history of possible exposure.

Diagnosis is done using a post-mortem direct fluorescence antibody test performed by a state-approved laboratory for rabies diagnosis. This means that the test can only be performed on dogs after they have died or been euthanized and in designated laboratories. (Refer to chapter- 7 for a list)

Treatment for Rabies in Dogs

If your dog has been vaccinated against rabies, your dog will receive a booster rabies vaccine. If anyone came into contact with the dog's saliva or was bitten by your dog, advise them to contact a physician immediately for treatment. Unfortunately, rabies is always fatal for unvaccinated animals, usually occurring within 7 to 10 days from when the initial symptoms began.

Once you have taken your dog to the veterinarian, disinfect any area the animal might have infected (especially with saliva) using a 1:32 dilution of household bleach solution to quickly inactivate the virus. Do not allow yourself to come into contact with your dog's saliva.

Rabies is a fatal virus. The best way to prevent the virus is to vaccinate your dog based on the schedule recommended by your veterinarian and local health department.

CHAPTER 10

How Do I keep My Dog Safe From Rabies?

Proper vaccination is the best and only way to keep you and your dog safe from Rabies.

There is no test that can be done on a living person or on an animal to diagnose if they are infected, and there is no treatment that can stop the disease once symptoms occur. Only when you are able to tell if you or your pet is infected with the virus, it is too late.

If your dog is not timely vaccinated against rabies and bites, gets bitten or has a wound of unknown origin that could possibly be a bite, the US law may require that pet be quarantined or even euthanized. This becomes necessary to keep other pets and people safe. These laws are different in different countries.

In India, we have no facility to quarantine rabies suspect animals and killing them by any means is unlawful.

Keeping your pets up-to-date with their rabies vaccines is absolutely essential and is mandated by law.

Here is what you should know about rabies vaccinations.

Recommended Rabies vaccination schedule for your dog

In most countries, the first dose of rabies vaccine is generally given to puppies at or before 16 weeks of age and the second, one year after the first vaccine. Then, that dog will be vaccinated every year or every three years depending on the state law and the vaccine used.

Your veterinarian is the best person to guide you for your rabies vaccination requirements.

You are supposed to maintain the vaccination record of your pet. A sample record is as follows:

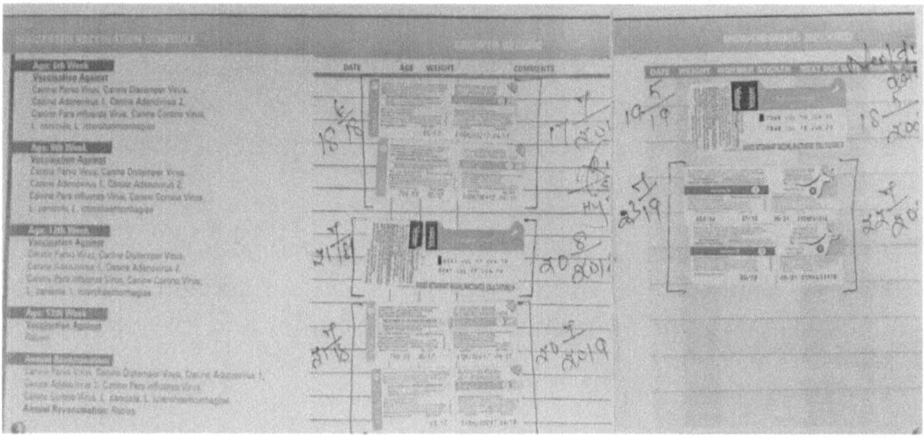

How Long Does a Rabies Vaccine Last?

This is a legal question as well as a medical one. There are rabies vaccines that are labeled as being effective for either one year or three years

Does my pet need Rabies boosters?

Over time, the effectiveness of the vaccine declines and that is why booster vaccines are required for your dog to stay protected.

Can a vaccinated dog get Rabies?

The rabies vaccine is extremely effective but at the same time we must not forget that no vaccine is 100% effective. There are a few reports of cases of vaccinated animals contracting rabies, because either vaccine was not perfect or dog's immune system did not respond well. As this is not possible to test immunity in every dog, owner is expected to take reasonable precautions, more so when rabies is endemic in that region.

The best prevention is to keep up to date on your dog's rabies vaccines and be protected yourself.

It is even better that street dogs are immunized by municipal authorities, panchayat authorities or NGOs. That will be a big step in direction of rabies elimination.

Relocating to a Different Country With a Pet

It can get challenging because of the complex pet import regulations in different countries. The paperwork and the health tests must be accurate and completed at the right time; failure to do so could result in your pet being denied entry or having to undergo more health tests or spending extra time in quarantine.

If you are planning to relocate internationally with your pet dog or cat, read at https://www.petraveller.com.au/blog/understanding-rabies-country-classification for a detailed travel itinerary and other pet travel advice.

CHAPTER 11 Can Rabies be Eliminated

Why does rabies still exist?

Approximately 90% of all reported rabies cases in the US are from wildlife. Wildlife species, primarily bats, raccoons, skunks, and foxes, act as reservoir for different variants of the rabies virus. This results in the general occurrence of rabies as wel outbreaks in animal population. The infected animal bites other animals and humans too before it dies.

Humans are a dead end as they do not bite others under usual circumstances. But other animals are not.

Rabies exists for all mammals including humans. It exists because all mammals which are capable of transferring rabies virus aren't vaccinated.

Attaining global eradication is the goal of anti-rabies organizations, but most see it as an aspiration, not a likely Achievement. This is not because the science is difficult, or the practical methods are unproven, but, like all public health problems, rabies control depends on large and continuing government action.

Medically, rabies is easy to prevent, in dogs and people.

Organizationally, the path to stopping rabies is well understood.

Eradication of canine Rabies in dog population, which is how human deaths drop to zero, requires a long-term commitment. To reach zero human deaths, the 120 countries, in which the disease is endemic would need huge money and act efficiently, now.

World Health Organization has announced a campaign to reduce human deaths from dog-transmitted rabies across the globe to zero by 2030.

It seems unlikely, looking at present state of affairs.

For this to become reality, we have to immunize every human being likely to come in contact with dogs, cats and practically any mammal. This will prevent human rabies; but animals will continue to suffer.

In fact every important public programs need strong political will which is not there in many governments.

Can Rabies be eliminated?

Difficult, as a big pool of rabies is among wild animals.

Rather, achieving the '**rabies free state'** can be the immediate goal. Our primary concern is saving human beings and animals around, pet as well as stray animals. Remember, many countries could achieve this goal.

Nature made many countries free of rabies as this virus never reached there. A union territory of India also has this natural advantage.

So are there countries that are free of rabies?

The following countries are currently recognized by the Canadian Food Inspection Agency as being free from rabies:

- Anguilla
- Antigua
- Australia
- Bahamas
- Barbados
- Bermuda
- Cayman Islands
- Fiji
- Finland
- Iceland
- Ireland (Republic of)
- Jamaica
- Japan
- New Zealand

- Norway
- Saint Kitts and Nevis
- Saint Lucia
- Saint Martin (Netherlands Antilles)
- Saint Pierre et Miquelon
- Saint Vincent and the Grenadines
- Sweden
- Turks and Caicos Islands
- United Kingdom (England, Scotland, Wales, Northern Ireland)
- Uruguay

Ref: Countries Recognized as Rabies Free for Domestic Cats and Dogs

What about stray animals in all these countries? Are they too rabies free in these countries?

In most, rabies never existed.

But if you remove rabies from the animals that come in human contact most of the times, you are safe.

Wild animals may have it and die once infected. It limits the pool of infection and its spread. Nature's way of disease control.

It can be managed by giving pre exposure prophylaxis in routine to people working with animals or exposed to animals in or around forests.

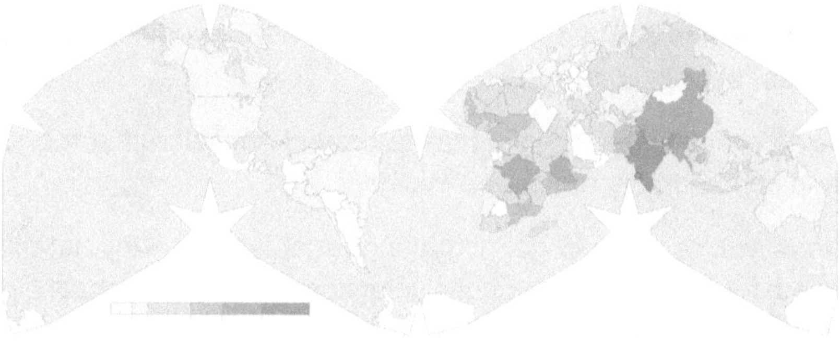

scale 0 patients --→20000 patients

By Jonathan Corum | Source: World Health Organization. Cahill-Keyes World Map projection by Gene Keyes

Rabies has been eliminated in dogs throughout much of **North America** and **Europe**.

India accounts for about a third of rabies deaths from dogs, but the disease is endemic in 120 countries.

Is rabies as fatal to animals as it is to humans?

Yes, rather more.

Most unprotected animals die fast.

Longer incubation period in humans gives a window for intervention and most human sufferers are saved by means of post exposure prophylaxis.

So if we somehow get rid of Rabies just like we got rid of small pox, will it eventually be extinct?

It is only possible when

1. All animals get vaccination or die with infection without being able to bite any more healthy individuals or animals
2. If they bite someone meanwhile and that person or animal is vaccinated in time or has PrEP.

If this becomes possible, virus will have no host and thus disease will be extinct.

How common is it for veterinarians to have themselves vaccinated for rabies, as a precaution?

This is as essential as using gloves to protect oneself rather more than that and is mandatory almost everywhere.

You know you're going to get bitten sooner or later, so why not obviate the need for the Immunoglobulin injection, which is probably pretty expensive and may be painful?

It is different in Australia as they have no rabies. They have VERY STRICT quarantine laws so there is only the remote chance of

Rabies usually by someone infected overseas (and comes here in the incubation period). Most of the animals known to transmit are carefully regulated in Zoos and are properly looked after. If an animal is imported or somebody takes it to Australia, it has to be quarantined.

Can animals get rabies if they're on an island?

They will not if there is no source of infection. All the dogs, cats and other mammals are not essentially carrying rabies virus. If no one has it, no one will have it.

Many countries or parts of countries are rabies free because of this natural advantage.

Union territory of Andaman & Nicobar and Lakshadweep are also free of rabies because of natural water barrier while rest of the country suffers rabies.

Oral rabies vaccine (for Animals)

There is an oral vaccination in pellet form which can be left out for wild animals to produce a herd immunity effect.

Oral Rabies Vaccination (ORV) programs have been used in many countries in an effort to control the spread of rabies and limit the risk of human contact with the rabies virus. ORV programs were initiated in Europe in the 1980s, Canada in 1985, and in the United States in 1990. ORV is a preventive measure to eradicate rabies in wild animal vectors of disease, mainly foxes, raccoons, raccoon dogs, coyotes and jackals, but also can be used for dogs in developing countries. ORV programs typically use edible baits to deliver the vaccine to targeted animals. ORV baits consist of a small packet containing the oral vaccine which is then either coated in a fishmeal paste or encased in a fishmeal-polymer block. When an animal bites into the bait, the packets burst and the vaccine is administered. Current research suggests that if adequate amounts of the vaccine are ingested, immunity to the virus should last for upwards of one year. By immunizing wild or stray animals, ORV programs work to create a buffer zone between the rabies virus and potential contact with humans, pets, or livestock.

Baits are usually distributed by aircraft to more efficiently cover large, rural regions. In order to place baits more precisely and to minimize human and pet contact with baits, however, they are distributed by hand in suburban or urban regions.

CHAPTER 12

Will the Problem of Rabies in India Ever be Solved?

Why are the Indian government and health organizations not serious about eradicating rabies from the country the way they are serious about other diseases, considering the fact that India is number one in the world for rabies cases?

Yes, the idea of a 'Rabies Free Nation' is quite pleasing.

Freeing a nation (or a geographical entity) from a germ/bacteria/virus calls for an astounding effort that is directed against desease. As long as the agent is tough at its survival qualities, it is much more difficult or impossible to remove it from its predilections.

Solution has to be practical, feasible and economical.

Rabies. 1) It survives in mammals; 2) Immunization effect in animals is not life-long. Just these two factors makes eradication difficult,, not economical and hence not feasible (in near future).

India is the number one in the world for number of disases because of its huge population. Rabies is one of them.

Eradication of rabies in India would involve vaccination of 25-30 million stray dogs. And even that is not completely fool proof as we have a large variety of wildlife which can transmit rabies, including bats.

We have to do this while managing many other health priorities like Polio, tuberculosis, HIV, dengue and malaria and now Corona. Rabies kills about 20,000 people a year in India. Tuberculosis kills about 220,000. We have about 100,000 cases of dengue every year and have 2.1 million people having HIV and now Corona is added.

There are a bunch of other diseases and disorders such as heart disorders, Diabetes, protein deficiency, cholera etc which affect significantly more number of people.

Whole health department is busy in tackling corona pandemic.

Rabies eradication, though important, falls far behind in the list of priorities.

World Health Organization has announced a campaign to reduce human deaths from dog-transmitted rabies across the globe to zero by 2030.

It seems unlikely, looking at present state of affairs.

For this to become reality, we have to immunize every human being likely to come in contact with dogs, cats and practically any mammal. This will prevent human rabies; but animals will continue to suffer.

In India, culling dogs is not allowed on humanitarian grounds. A 2001 Indian law details how dogs should be humanely caught, housed, Sterilized and released back onto the street. Experts say culling is not very effective method.

At least half of the patients with rabies are bitten by pet dogs.

So the authorities turn to vaccinating not just the human population, but the dogs as well.

If 70% of the dog population was vaccinated, that would be enough to contain the spread of the virus. According to the 2015 PLOS study, by 2010 India had vaccinated just 15% of its dogs.

And vaccinations alone are not enough. The dogs must also be sterilized to make sure new animals – potential reservoirs for the virus – aren't introduced into the community.

All said and done, India has no national or state-wide plans in effect to make this happen.

Pre-exposure immunization of millions of humans with ARV seems very difficult and immunizing all dogs and cats (and many more animals) is practically impossible.

Human rabies can be prevented as many countries did but not the rabies as a whole.

CHAPTER 13

Goa Is Free of Human Rabies for 3 Years. What is Their Success Story?

By **Nandita Subbarao** on Quora with inputs from **James Gorman** in NewYork Times (July 22, 2019)

Goa has had an NGO called Mission Rabies active there for a few years now. Mission Rabies is a part of World Veterinary Services (WVS), a reputed NGO headquartered in the UK.

Mission Rabies embarked on a panchayat-by-panchayat census by sending teams of people on two-wheelers. This is effective in navigating narrow or bad roads. Also, the crew is able to get close, even befriend the dog, and quickly give it the anti-rabies shot. After the two-wheeler team covers whatever it can in the first couple of days (typically about half the dogs), a van goes to the area, and the catchers use nets to catch and vaccinate the rest (and release them immediately). You can read about the statistics at http://www.missionrabies.com/projects/india/. In fact, they even vaccinate the *pet* dogs they find, with the permission of the owner.

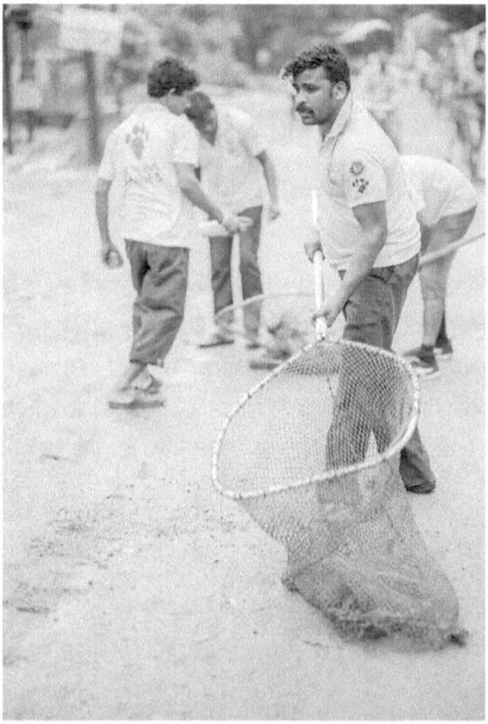

A quick twist of a net immobilizes, restrains and calms a captured dog so that it can be vaccinated and released quickly.

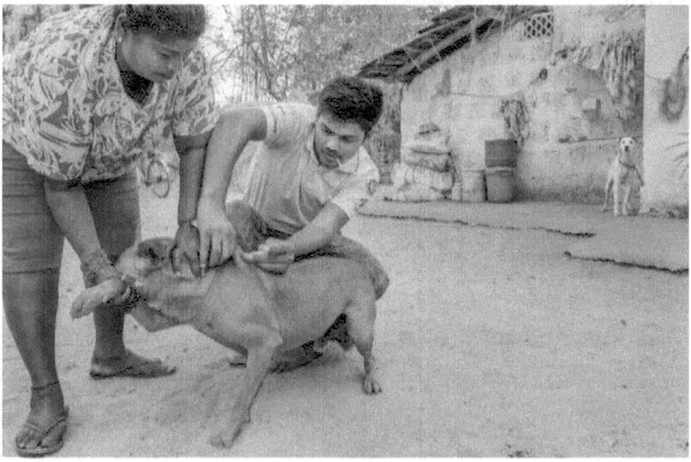

Pet dogs may also roam free, but are often easily approached and held by owner to be vaccinated.

They have been doing this every year, so we can assume that most of the dogs are now vaccinated. They also send volunteers to schools, to sensitize and condition children on the role that dogs play in the environment, how to behave with them, etc.

Neutering is not a part of their agenda; there are other NGOs that focus on this.

- Mission Rabies has also set up a 24-hour hotline. a number that local residents could call to report rabid dog sightings. This allowed their team to locate and remove rabid dogs, and complete a ring vaccination of 200-300 at-risk dogs in the area, stopping the spread of the disease in its tracks.

People can call in to report a dog bite, where a counselor asks for details. The victim and the biting dog are kept under observation.

Communication is also very important — the government and Mission Rabies together ensure that the message reaches every panchayat.

What they have done is commendable. A structured approach (with excellent communication) is needed in every ward and every village. Goa and Mission Rabies have led the way.

Ryan M. Wallace, a veterinarian who heads the rabies epidemiology unit at the Centers for Disease Control and Prevention in Atlanta and who has collaborated with Mission Rabies in Haiti, said its effort in Goa is "one of the most successful programs in lower/middle income countries that I have seen in a decade."

Mission Rabies estimates the vaccination cost per dog, including salaries and other costs, at $2.50, far lower than the cost of treating humans, which involves not only a more expensive vaccine, but also potential hospital stays. By that accounting, every dog in India could theoretically be vaccinated for under $90 million. India now spends $490 million a year on post-bite treatment, Dr. Gibson estimated.

History:

2013- big launch, 61,143 dogs vaccinated in just 1 month!

In 2014: sterilised 20,400 dogs across Goa in a 6 month long campaign.

Set up out Rabies hotline.

2015 was a HUGE year in India, smashing previous vaccination records, delivering 94,753 rabies vaccinations!

The end of 2016 brought about the start of a Mission Rabies and WVS (Worldwide Veterinary Service) synergistic partnership in Goa.

There was a clear decline in human rabies deaths in Goa from 17 in 2014, 5 in 2015 and only 1 in 2016!

There have gradually been fewer cases of bites, and there was no human rabies death in 2018 and probably 2019 too — see Rabies Kills Tens of Thousands Yearly. Vaccinating Dogs Could Stop It..

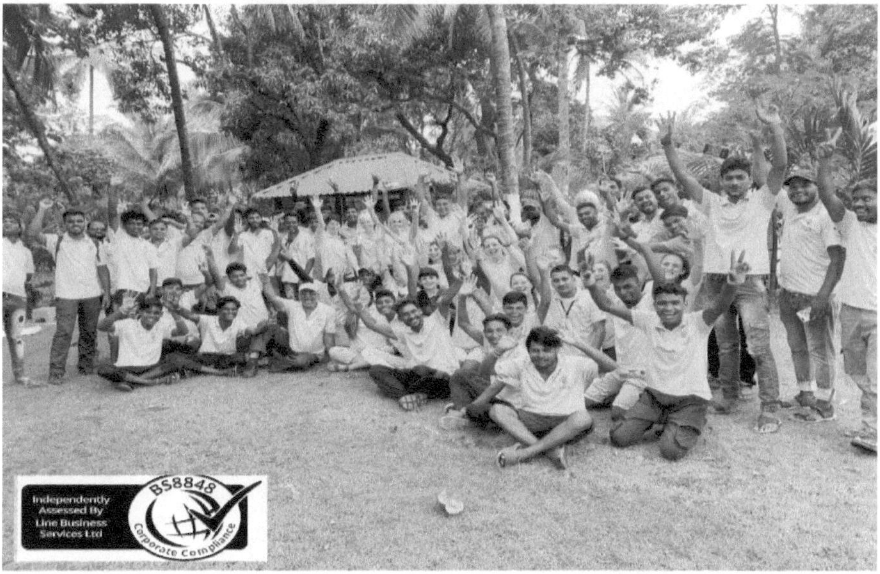

Success story of Ranchi, Jharkhnd

This is similar to success story of Goa.

This is the story of **empowering communities** with the knowledge that they need to protect themselves from rabies.

Mass canine vaccination will rid an area of rabies, but this takes time during which communities remain at risk – whilst they work to eliminate the disease for good, education helps save lives.

Delivered life-saving lessons to children:

Education Officers delivered rabies prevention lessons to children – the group most at risk of being infected by the deadly disease and taught students about rabies, dog bite prevention and lifesaving first aid – knowledge that could one day save their lives or that of a loved one.

Gaining insight to save lives:

With greater insight, we can have a greater impact.

That's why Mission Rabies education teams run focus groups in the areas where they vaccinate dogs. It helps them better appreciate the community's understanding of and attitudes towards rabies. They use this knowledge to improve their programs and save more lives.

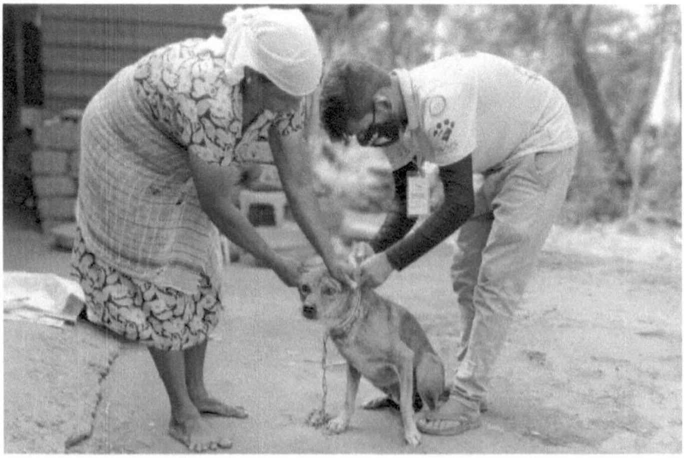

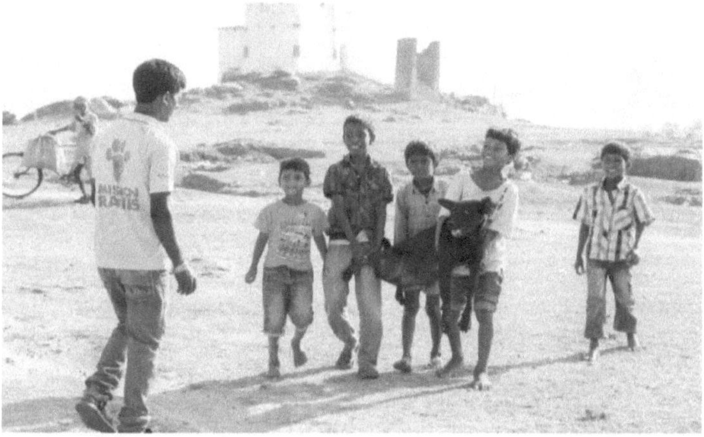

Children bringing their friendly dog for vaccination.

Helping Organisation for People, Environment and Animal Trust (**HOPE & Animal Trust**) has been providing animal welfare services in Ranchi and Varanasi for more than 10 years. They care for thousands of stray animals each year treating for severe wounds, operating to control the population and finding new forever homes.

Ranchi Celebrated Rabies Free 2017!

In India, a child dies every minute from rabies and in Jharkhand State, around 50 lives are lost each year to this 100% vaccine-preventable disease. Besides the huge cost to human life, rabies costs the Indian economy over Rs.16.6 crore per year. These truly concerning statistics were behind the decision for Dogs Trust-sponsored Mission Rabies, working with Ranchi NGO, HOPE & Animal Trust, to join hands with Ranchi Municipal Corporation and the Animal Husbandry Department of Jharkhand Government, to work towards eliminating the threat of this terrible disease.

Key Facts from Ranchi: Total vaccinations in 2017 – 18 – 28,167, 10,774 dogs sterilised, Mean vaccination coverage was 72%, 80% of adult roaming dogs in the Ranchi are neutered, 138 Dogs were Euthanised ü 181 Dogs have been treated and released back healthy.

Varanasi also seen replica of the Ranchi Program

CHAPTER

14 Rabies Elimination: More Interesting Information From Goa and Other Places

Rabies perfectly illustrates the concept of "one health," the idea that the health of human and animal populations is necessarily tied together. Wherever there are people in the world, there are dogs. If dogs are suffering and dying from rabies, humans will also suffer and die. In essence, if you save dogs, you save humans.

The consensus among rabies experts is that if the level of vaccination in the dog population can be kept at 70 percent over a period of seven years, the variant of the rabies virus that thrives in dog populations will disappear.

Effective vaccination depends not only on technical tools but also on an understanding of dog-human relations. Who owns or cares for dogs in any given community? And how much control do the humans have over the dog population?

In countries where dogs have become leash-bound pets, like the United States and Western Europe, canine rabies has been eliminated. The result of this is that there are 1 to 3 deaths a year, that too, caused by contact with bats, dog bites outside the country or bites from other animals, like raccoons. In most of the Americas, national governments have political will and devoted enough budget to vaccinate the vast majority of dogs every year, so even in countries where the disease is not eliminated, deaths are rare.

In Africa, where thousands of people die from rabies each year, most dogs, even if they are in streets, are owned by families, and vaccination drives can concentrate on the owners, who will bring them to vaccination locations.

India is different. Street dogs and people in India often have a kind of understanding. The dogs aren't wild, but they aren't owned either. Free-roaming dogs are often supported by the community but no one owns them. Nobody decides when and where they live, eat or mate. Lock-down due to Corona has been a very difficult period for these stray dogs. They did not find food outside eateries and no one fed them in streets.

There are about 30 to 35 million dogs in India, compared with 90 million dogs in the United States. India is 1/3 the size of the United States geographically, and 3 times the size in population. This means that the number of dogs per acre or city block is about the same and the number of dogs per person far less. The difference is that in India, the dogs are mostly outside; in the United States, they are mostly indoors.

Rabies campaigns in other countries often involve getting owners to bring dogs to central vaccination points, but that poses problems in India, because of the lack of individual ownership. The answer, according to Mission Rabies, is to send out teams to find and vaccinate street dogs, using a variety of techniques with about 40 percent requiring capture by nets.

The Mission Rabies program has three aspects: vaccination, education and data gathering.

At the heart of the plan is a Smartphone app that allows the vaccination teams to track their GPS-monitored progress through a neighborhood on a map as they move from street to street. Team leaders can easily see each day's progress. And the accumulated data helps set the next day's plan and provide information for analysis. The C.D.C., which advises the Haitian government, used the app there and achieved an increase in dogs vaccinated to 76 percent from 40 percent.

Cost effectiveness of immunizing dogs: Mission Rabies estimates the vaccination cost per dog, including salaries and other costs, at $2.50, that is far lower than the cost of treating humans, which involves not only a more expensive vaccine, but also potential hospital stays. By that accounting, all the dogs in India could theoretically be vaccinated for under $90 million. India now spends $490 million a year on post-bite treatment, Dr. Gibson estimated.

It may be said that Goa's project is too small a model to be replicated at a large scale.

Applying the Goa project's methods on a larger scale would require at least one technical piece that is missing — **an oral vaccine**. Western Europe eradicated rabies in foxes by dropping baits with oral vaccines, beginning in 1990 when rabies was widespread and lasting more than 20 years.

The oral vaccine has also been tested in dogs in Haiti and other countries with success. And Dr. Gibson has run tests to show how the oral vaccine can reduce the number of people needed to reach hard-to-vaccinate dogs. Many dogs now caught in nets might approach hand-tossed bait.

The parent organization of Mission Rabies does include programs that **train vets and sterilize dogs**. And population control of dogs, through sterilization (with vaccination), is the approach preferred by Humane Society International.

> The WHO wants to eliminate Rabies in Asia by 2020. But how, when India accounts for more than one third of the world's total Rabies deaths?
>
> – *Mary-Rose Abraham reports.*

This is part of an ongoing – and some say uphill – battle to eliminate rabies from India. Around 59,000 people die from rabies every year, according to a 2015 study published in PLOS Neglected Tropical Diseases. The overwhelming majority are in Asia and Africa: India alone accounts for 20,847 deaths; more than one-third of the world's total, giving it the highest incidence of rabies globally.

The World Health Organization (WHO) wants to eliminate rabies from the South-East Asia region by the year 2020. It is a goal that India is unlikely to meet, public health experts say.

With rabies, the country doesn't even know the extent of the disease. There is no requirement for doctors to report human infections, and no information on how widespread it might be among animals. In 2014, India's government said it would set up a national rabies control programme, but at the time of writing it has only launched a pilot project in the northern state of Haryana to advice on managing the problem nationwide.

Meanwhile, the government leaves it to the local city authorities to carry out programmes for vaccinating stray dogs on the street. Most deal with the problem by hiring NGOs like CUPA. That leaves rural areas, where rabies strikes hardest, all but ignored.

About one in 143 Indians is bitten by a dog at some point in their lives.

The WHO recommends pre-exposure vaccinations for everyone in rabies-endemic countries. India's own Academy of Pediatrics also recommends children are vaccinated, but relatively few are ever immunized. People may not realize the extent of the danger – and the benefit of vaccination.

To truly eliminate rabies from India, animal health is the key, yet the extent of rabies infection in the country's animals remains a mystery.

If You Wish to Read Further

https://apps.who.int/iris/bitstream/handle/10665/272364/9789241210218-eng.pdf

WHO: Control and elimination strategies

www.who.int/rabies/control/en

World Health Organization. Rabies vaccines: WHO Position Paper, April 2018 Recommendations.

Vaccine. 2018;36:5500-3.

WHO | The Rabies Elimination Program of Bangladesh

www.who.int/neglected_diseases/news/Bangladesh.

https://www.petraveller.com.au/blog/understanding-rabies-country-classification

http://www.missionrabies.com/projects/india/

World Health Organization. Rabies vaccines: WHO Position Paper, April 2018 Recommendations. Vaccine. 2018;36:5500-3

National Rabies Control Programme (of India)

National Guidelines on Rabies Prophylaxis revised after extensive expert consultations after newly endorsed WHO recommendations for Rabies prophylaxis in WHO TRS 1012.

NATIONAL CENTRE FOR DISEASE CONTROL hp://www.ncdc.gov.in 2015

Indian Journal of Medical Ethics CASE STUDY using a modified rabies immunoglobulin protocol in

a crisis of unavailability: Ethical and practical challenges Omesh Kumar Bharti DOI:

https://doi.org/10.20529/IJME.2019.022

Zero by 30: the global strategic plan to end human deaths from dog-mediated rabies by 2030

www.ingramcontent.com/pod-product-compliance
Lightning Source LLC
Chambersburg PA
CBHW020913180526
45163CB00007B/2713